This book belongs to...

Disclaimer

The contents of this book are for information only and are intended to assist readers in identifying symptoms and conditions they may be experiencing. This book is not intended to be a substitute for obtaining proper medical advice and must not be relied upon in this way. Always consult a qualified doctor or health practitioner. The author and publisher do not accept responsibility for illness arising out of the failure to seek medical advice from a doctor. In the event that you use any of the information in this book for yourself or your family or friends, the author and the publisher assume no responsibility for your actions.

Copyright © Dr Libby Weaver, 2016

PUBLISHED BY Little Green Frog Publishing Pty Ltd
www.littlegreenfrogpublishing.com

Art direction and publication design:
Stephanie Antill

Photography:
Sabine Bannard

ISBN: 978-0-473-36088-7

Printed in China

Dr Libby's

Women's Wellness Wisdom

WHAT EVERY WOMAN NEEDS TO KNOW

Dr Libby Weaver

CONGRATULATIONS ON PURCHASING

Women's Wellness Wisdom

The science and understanding of the impact that nutrition and lifestyle choices have on our bodies is constantly changing as colleagues in the research world continue to make breakthroughs.

By purchasing this book you qualify to become a Registered Reader. Our aim with this is to ensure that we are able to keep you abreast of the latest developments in health and wellbeing, as well as provide you with a touch point to continue to motivate you to achieve the goals you desire for your health and body.

Please become a Registered Reader by visiting:
www.drlibby.com/registered-reader

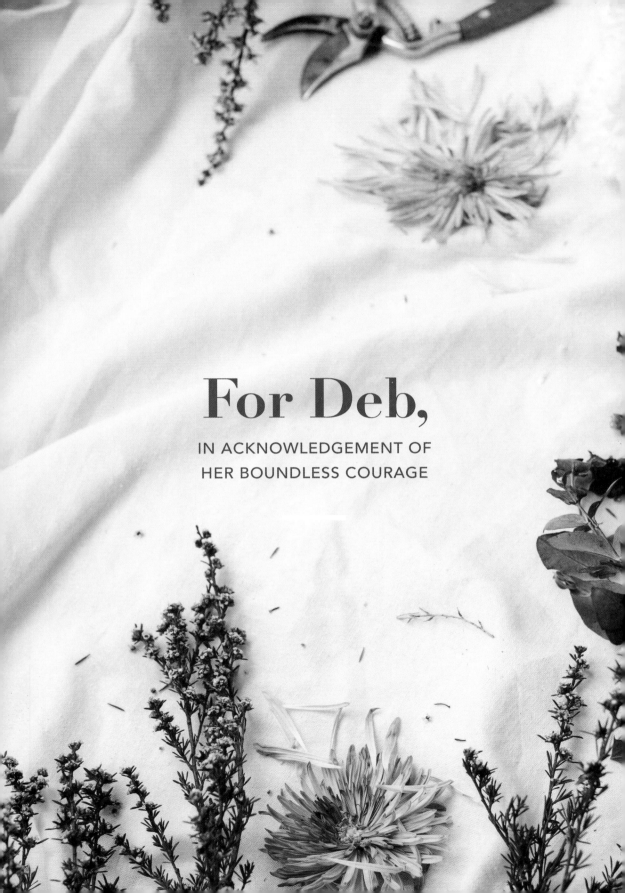

For Deb,

IN ACKNOWLEDGEMENT OF
HER BOUNDLESS COURAGE

CONTENTS

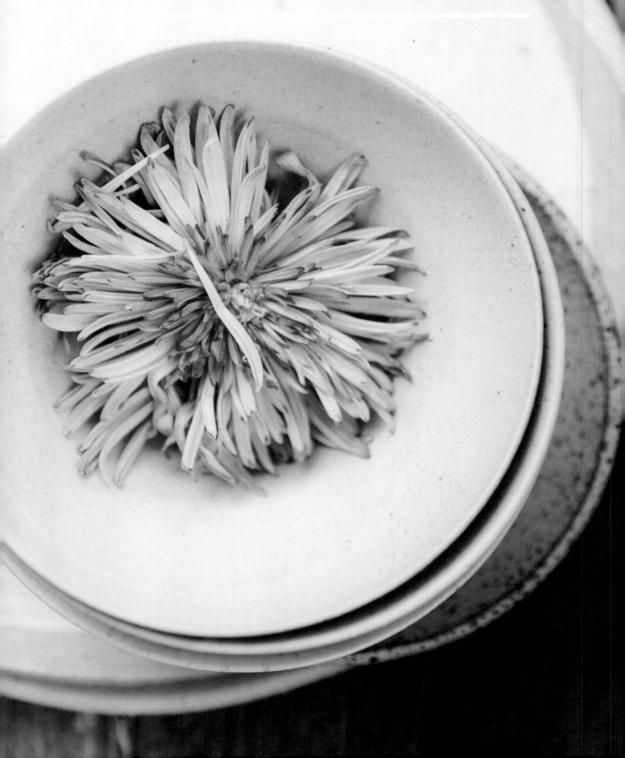

EAT

BODY

CONTENTS

CONTENTS

MIND

WORLD

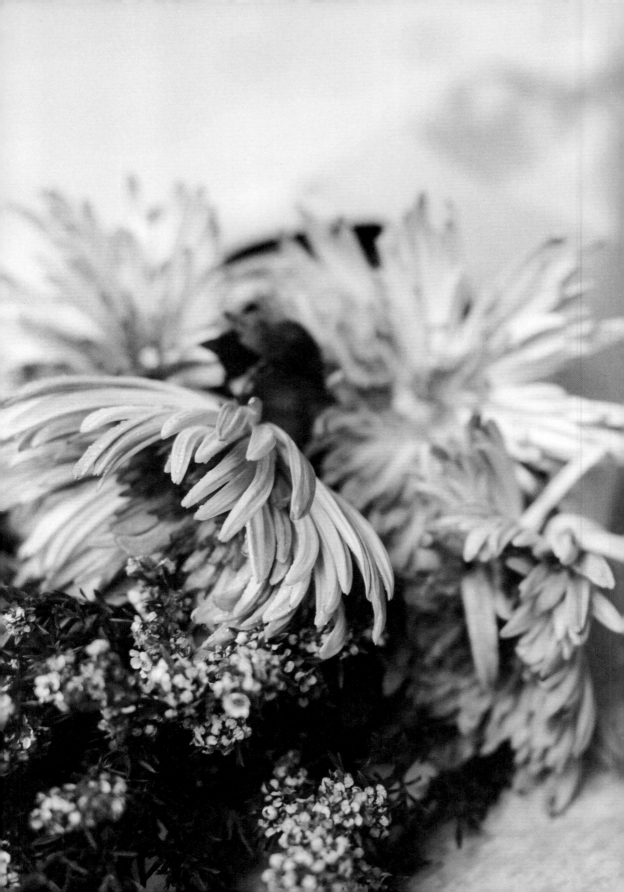

My mission is to educate and inspire, enhancing people's health and happiness, igniting a ripple effect that transforms the world.

Dr Libby Weaver

Introduction

Welcome to a new way of experiencing your health.
My hope for this book is that it will offer you an understanding of the inner workings of your body as well as some simple strategies to help you feel your best. When we step up and take care of ourselves, it doesn't just impact on us, it affects everyone around us. We all want to experience meaningful lives. We want to contribute.
Yet this can become more and more challenging, the less energy and the more debilitating, poor health symptoms we have. Sadly, when a symptom doesn't make us stay home from work, we often do nothing about it, until the dysfunction that led to the symptoms occurring in the first place goes further and something potentially more sinister has unfolded. I want this book to teach you that your body is your most insightful barometer, offering you feedback about your choices. I am hopeful that this book will help you to make more nourishing choices for your body, mind and soul.

I am also hopeful that this book will offer you simple tools that foster an even healthier and happier life, helping you to appreciate even more deeply how miraculous your body truly is and the gift that you are to the world.

You may (I believe, incorrectly) assume that you need more motivation to be healthy. Yet what is more likely is that you need to get back in touch with how precious you are and treat yourself accordingly.

If that sounds wishy-washy then try this on instead:
if you knew who you truly are, you would be in awe of yourself,
and you would never do half of the things you currently do to
yourself. It's time to make better choices,
because you know you are worth taking care of.

Yet it's not only about what you get — better health and energy,
for example — it's also about who you become through the
process of taking better care of yourself, and I have witnessed,
in thousands of people, that taking better care of their health can
be a doorway to so much more opening up in their lives.

My style is never to instruct or boss you around, or to lead you
to feel deprived. I want you to understand the inner workings
of your body and deeply appreciate them. You inherently
make more nourishing choices from this place.

My work has also never just been about the individual; in fact,
I am obsessed with the ripple effect on others and the planet,
which every choice we make generates. You will hear these
sentiments echoed throughout these pages, encouraging you,
too, to think big, to look beyond your immediate surroundings.
We must never be too busy for that.

I hope this book also offers a sense a spaciousness in your life,
for even though what we must attend to each day may not
change, how we approach it can. And the more space we
perceive, the more ease and grace flows in our lives,
with less stress and more trust.

With much warmth,

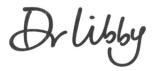

EA

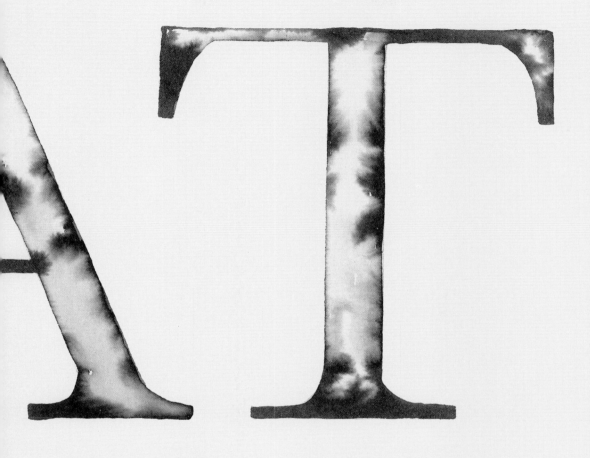

The way you eat is the most basic way you demonstrate care for yourself. There is nothing in this world that replaces a highly nourishing way of eating. There is nothing that can burn off a lousy way of eating. Consuming whole, real-food is the basis of exceptional health. I have never witnessed long-term sustained change come from deprivation. It always begins with kindness. Be kind to yourself, including through the foods you eat.

food

WHY WHAT WE EAT MATTERS

Have you ever considered that what you eat actually becomes part of you? Food offers us far more than just energy and nutrients. It has the capacity to be our most powerful medicine or to actively take away from our health. There is nothing in the world that can replace a highly nutritious way of eating. Nothing. No amount of exercise can burn off the effects of a poor-quality way of eating. It is, after all, nutrients that keep us alive.

NUTRIENTS

Even though it is nutrients that keep us alive, I feel most people don't hear enough about their importance. An adult's body is made up of about 50 trillion cells. That is a number that can go over our head with its enormity, as we tend to hear the word "trillion" on the news regularly, usually in reference to US debt, and as a result it can seem to be much smaller than it is. So I will use time as an example to demonstrate the enormity of 1 trillion, let alone 50 trillion. One million seconds ago was 12 days ago. One billion seconds ago was 32 years ago, but 1 trillion seconds ago was 32,000 years ago. And we are made up of about 50 trillion cells.

Imagine you are made up of 50 trillion little tiny circles that all want to talk to each other, and the only way that they can communicate is when there are nutrients present. Imagine, then, what happens when people aren't getting adequate nutrients for some of the very basic processes, let alone for optimal health, as I believe is the case.

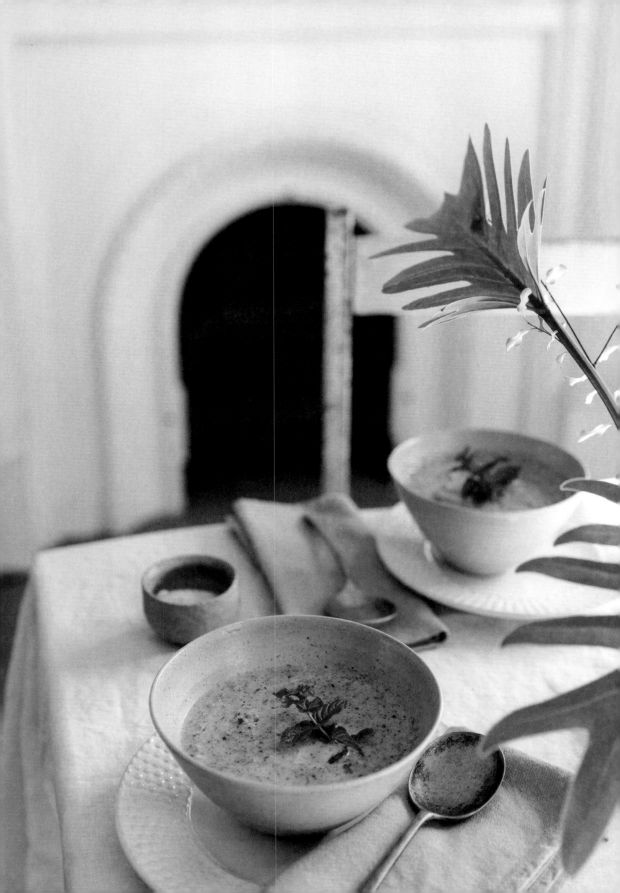

The cells of the body don't live forever. They are always in a cycle of replication, repair and death. Some cells turn over faster than others. For example, eye cells replicate quickly, whereas the bones do so slowly. Our whole outer layer of skin is replaced every 28 days. However, the health of the next generation of cells is dependent on the information they pick up on in their environment. And what's in their environment? Either plenty of nutrients or a lack of nutrients, with one or many lacking. There are also hormones at work — and at this point in the book, we will divide them into the categories of love and fear, for simplicity's sake — which are activated when we feel loving, appreciative feelings, and also when we feel fearful. The health and quality of each new cell is powerfully influenced by this information.

When I was doing my undergraduate studies in nutrition and dietetics, as well as during my PhD in biochemistry, I had the biochemical pathways of the human body mapped out on large pieces of paper, stuck to my bedroom walls. It was the only way I was ever going to learn them. When you see the body mapped out like this, you develop a deep appreciation for the critical role nutrients play in life itself. Every second there are billions of biochemical reactions taking place. What that means is that substance X has to be turned into substance Y, and for that to occur perhaps you need magnesium and vitamin B6. Without one or both of these nutrients the reaction cannot occur efficiently, and so substance X accumulates and you miss out on substance Y. And maybe if substance X accumulates it behaves more like a problem — a toxin — something your body will need to get rid of, and perhaps you need substance Y to sleep restoratively, or to create the hormones that allow you to feel happy, or for you to be able to access body fat and burn it as a fuel.

When you see the body mapped out like this, you don't just develop a deep appreciation for the critical role that nutrients play in health, but you also get a deep appreciation for the absolute miracle that we are. If you knew who you truly are, you would be in awe of yourself. However, too few people live their lives in touch with that, and therefore don't treat themselves accordingly.

YOUR ROLE

Due to the incredible advances of Western medicine, we are going to continue to live longer and longer. We are so fortunate to live in a time where there is such extraordinary emergency medicine available to us. Yet, in reality, are we living too short and dying too long? This is an important question to ponder; for what I care about is the quality of your life. Today, as well as in the later part of your life, you want to be able to bend over and do up your own shoelaces. Imagine what life would be like if you had to rely on someone else to do this? How would your once-independent self feel? You don't want this to happen because your tummy has grown too large for you to be able to reach your feet, and so in later years you sit back and wish you had changed the way you had eaten earlier. You don't want to not be able to reach your feet because you have led a sedentary lifestyle and in later years your spine is relatively inflexible and you can't bend to reach your feet. You don't want that to occur. So the ways you eat, drink, move, sleep, think, breathe, believe and perceive don't just impact on how you feel, function and look today — they are going to influence how you feel, function and look in the future. And the power to change all of that is in your hands — and in your hands only. Let that empower you.

The way you feed yourself is the most basic, most fundamental way you demonstrate care for yourself. It is time to stop dieting and start nourishing. It is time to stop counting calories if you do; if you need to count anything, count nutrients and amp them up, and count synthetic substances and omit them. You will see why and how throughout the pages of this book. Remember, it is nutrients that keep us alive.

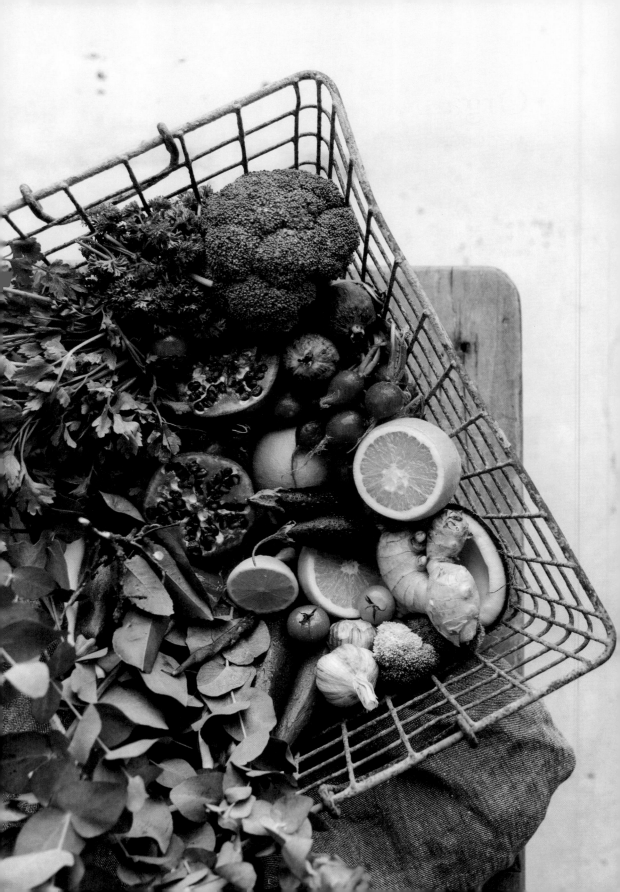

Organic

WHY ORGANIC FOOD MATTERS

Organic produce is labelled "certified organic" when it has been grown, raised, harvested and packaged without the use of potentially harmful chemicals, such as fertilizers, pesticides, insecticides, growth hormones and antibiotics. "Certified organic" also means that the produce has not been genetically modified. When we choose organic, we not only look after the health of our body systems, biochemical pathways and immune system, but also the health of our family, the health of the soil, and the health of the planet. Everyone benefits.

THE GOOD NEWS

The best way to get organic produce into how you eat is to grow it yourself. However, if that is not an option, try your local farmers' market, or search the internet for a company that delivers organic produce to your door. Even on some of the smallest apartment balconies I have stood on, I have seen an abundance of herbs in pots that nourish that family. There are also plots of land you can rent or hire on the outskirts of many cities these days, offering city dwellers who may not have much land the opportunity to harvest their own plot. The people with land will grow the vegetables you and your family like to eat, and you visit on the weekend and harvest what is grown. Yet another win-win for all involved.

THE BAD NEWS

The worldwide debate on the impact of conventional farming practices on soil fertility is getting a lot of attention. And rightly so, as many people are starting to take heed of ecologists' warnings about the impact of poor-quality soil on all life. More and more people are also discovering for themselves that maintenance of soil fertility is critical to the sustainability of the food supply.

In conventional farming practices, soils are used over and over and over again, usually without nutrient-dense replenishment. Every time a crop of vegetables, for example, is grown, it draws the nutrients out of the soil and into itself. The plant uses the nutrients to grow. Then we get the benefits of those nutrients when we eat that food. But if the nutrients aren't replaced, or there is no crop rotation, the soils are stripped of their minerals. Farmers then periodically saturate their crops with unnatural chemical fertilizers. I refer to them as "unnatural" for many reasons, one of which is that they don't contain the range of nutrients essential for life. They are primarily made up of three nutrients: nitrogen, phosphorus and potassium. This means that there are 52 nutrients missing.

Sadly, the impact of conventional farming methods doesn't end there. With poor soil health comes poor plant health, and when plants have lost their ability to defend themselves against pests, the pests come. Hence, the subsequent application of pesticides, herbicides and fungicides. That's how it happens. That's one of the ways and reasons pesticides have infiltrated our food supply. It all starts with the health of the soil. Poor soil health leads to poor plant health. This leads to the food supply being contaminated with substances that are potentially problematic to human health, plus the food is deficient in nutrients, as they are lacking in the soil. So our bodies can end up toxic and deficient.

When we choose organic, we not only look after the health of our body systems and biochemical pathways, but also the health of our family, the health of the soil, and the health of the planet.

Over the short term these nutrient deficiencies tend to manifest in us as lousy energy, body aches, joint pain, failing eyesight, and thousands of other scenarios that people are encouraged to simply accept as part of aging. Over the long term, nutrient deficiencies contribute to major illnesses, such as numerous cancers, heart disease and type 2 diabetes, to name but a few.

WHERE DO WE GO FROM HERE?

As Rachel Carson so insightfully wrote in 1962: "If we are going to live so intimately with these chemicals … taking them into the very marrow of our bones — we had better know something about their nature and their power." More than five decades later, we know more of their power, but we still have much to learn. It is time that that we break the cycle of weed-resistance that keeps farmers on a pesticide treadmill, and phase out their reliance on potentially health-harming herbicides.

Sometimes it takes a health crisis to wake you up to make changes to your lifestyle choices, or at least to investigate them. And that's what I see more and more people doing when it comes to their exposure to potentially problematic substances. What I am referring to here are the pesticides and herbicides with which conventional produce is sprayed, and the synthetic chemicals with which people clean their homes and wash their clothes, as well as put on their skin. We are fortunate to live in a world where we have access to alternatives.

On 20 March 2015, scientists from 11 countries convened by the World Health Organization's (WHO) International Agency for Research on Cancer released their unanimous conclusions about the world's most used herbicide: glyphosate. In a paper that would be published in *The Lancet Oncology*, one of the most prestigious medical journals in the world, the experts concluded that the herbicide is "probably carcinogenic to humans". Yes, you read that right: the most widely used herbicide in the world probably causes cancer in humans. Barely used on US farm land as recently as 1992, by 2012 an estimated 250 million pounds (about 113 million kilograms) were being used. Unfortunately, I was unable to obtain statistics related to the use Down Under, but it is likely to be comparable given similar agricultural practices.

Then there's this: an international group of scientists, led by a team at the University of Canterbury in New Zealand, found that exposure to some formulations of glyphosate and other common herbicides can lead to antibiotic resistance in bacteria, including resistance to ciprofloxacin, which is commonly used in human medicine. This is deeply concerning, so it is well worth considering where and how you can begin to decrease your exposure to these potentially problematic substances.

If you feel that cost is a barrier to what I fondly refer to as 'low-tox' choices, explore your priorities and see if there is flexibility there. When funds were very tight for me, I didn't buy any new clothes or shoes for four years unless they cost less than five dollars (ie, op-shop). That's how much eating organic food, cleaning with low-tox products and using organic skincare meant to me.

Despite all of our accomplishments in the world, we owe our existence to a 30-centimetre layer of topsoil and the fact that it rains. It is estimated that more than 3 billion tons of topsoil is eroded from US farmlands each year, and soil is eroding seven times faster than it is being built up naturally. In organic farming, soil is the foundation of the food chain, and it is therefore critically important to support organic and sustainable agriculture sooner rather than later for the health of people and the planet. From a health perspective, when we choose organics we not only look after the health of our own body and immune system but, as I said at the beginning, also the health of our family, the health of our soil, and the health of our planet. So everyone wins.

YOUR CHOICES

When it comes to pesticides, we really are guinea pigs with regards to the long-term consumption of these substances. The reason your store-bought apple looks so perfect is because it has been sprayed to make it that way. Even though we cannot see or taste the chemicals on its skin, they are there. Pesticides have to be tested before they can be used on food for human consumption. However, they are often tested for such a short length of time that I do not believe we can compare tests done over, say, a six-month period, to being exposed to these things over an entire lifetime. It is also not possible to test what happens when all of the chemicals are mixed and then combined inside our bodies every day when we eat conventionally grown produce.

Fresh food the way it comes in Nature is an incredibly important part of our diets, and I encourage you to choose organic produce whenever you can. Also, think about the way you eat the food. We peel a banana. It may have been sprayed, but how much gets through the skin? We don't know, but it would seem reasonable to assume that there would be less chemical residue in the flesh (inside) of a banana than on the skin. So perhaps choosing a conventionally grown banana is not too bad. Yet when it comes to an apple, we usually eat the whole fruit. So in this case you would be better to choose an organic (or biodynamically grown) apple wherever possible.

Contemplate this: organic food is the true cost of food. I once started and ran an organic café.

Once a week, a local farmer delivered fresh greens picked that morning from his biodynamic farm. I always set aside some time on the day of his delivery to chat with him, as he always had wonderful tales to tell of life on his farm. One day, when I asked him how he was, his reply was along the lines of "not so good".

> *Fresh food the way it comes in Nature is an incredibly important part of our diets, and I encourage you to choose organic produce whenever you can.*

When I enquired further, he went on to tell me that snails had invaded his broccoli patch virtually overnight.

When I paused to consider this, I realized that if they took hold a portion of this man's

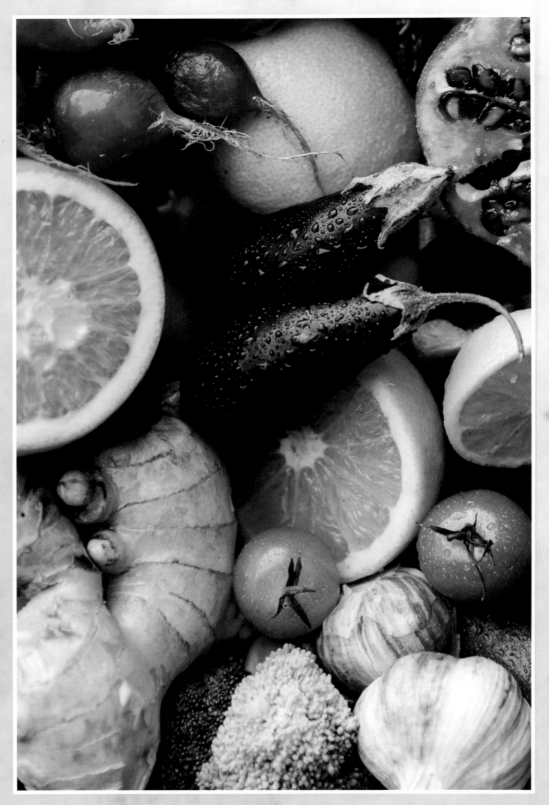

meagre livelihood would be lost. So I asked him how he deals with snails on his broccoli, given that his farming principles do not involve spraying the patch to get rid of the invaders (which would have taken less than 30 minutes to do). My farmer friend went on to tell me that snails lose their "stick", their ability to suction onto things, in salty water. So he made up a bottle of salt and water, and then spent two days, crouched down on all fours, crawling between his broccoli plants, squirting saline water up under the leaves and florets. Not only that, he didn't kill the snails, but instead collected them in a bucket and fed them to the chickens — "to keep them in the food chain", as he so delightfully put it.

Think about each of these scenarios. Spray the entire crop in under 30 minutes versus crawling around on your haunches for two days. For me, that illustrates precisely why organic and biodynamic food costs more: it reflects the real cost of food. This is in addition to its having a greater nutritional value, not to mention what is left out by way of potentially problematic chemicals. The more of us who choose organic produce, the cheaper it will become. The more we demand organic and say no to pesticides, the more organics will have to be supplied. I know I am on my soapbox, and I really do want to remain real and practical with the advice I offer. So, in simple terms, choose organic food whenever you can.

If organic food is unavailable in your area, or it is too costly for you to buy, try this solution to remove pesticides. Pesticides tend to be fat-soluble, and so general washing to get rid of dirt and germs does not remove them. To clean food of both dirt and pesticides at the same time, fill your sink with three parts water to one part vinegar, and wash your fruits and vegetables. Then rinse them in fresh water, pat them dry and store them for use. Do what is practical for you. And then stretch a little.

Cost

EATING REAL FOOD ON A BUDGET

A common reason people often give for not eating whole, real-foods is because they perceive these foods as a lot more expensive than packaged or processed food, or consider that eating this way is not sustainable for most families.

HERE ARE SOME IDEAS TO HELP MAKE EATING WHOLEFOODS EASIER ON THE POCKET:

Eat seasonally

Buying and eating only in-season produce is not only good for your health, but it's also beneficial for your wallet. Fruit and vegetables grown in season are more likely to have been grown outside in natural conditions, where the plants are able to soak up and transform more nutrients. Also, seasonal food doesn't need to be shipped from other countries, ensuring fresher food (more nutrients) and cutting out the cost of travel.

Buy local

Buy local produce where possible. Not only does it support local farmers in your community, but you can often save money on produce as the shipping costs are eliminated from the price of the food. When buying from local farmers' markets, it is often possible to find spray-free or organic food for the same price as conventional produce.

Reduce portion sizes

Many people are eating portion sizes that are simply too big. Reduce your portion size by a quarter and see how you feel. Most people will find that they feel satisfied with less, and avoid the over-full feeling that so many people end their day with.

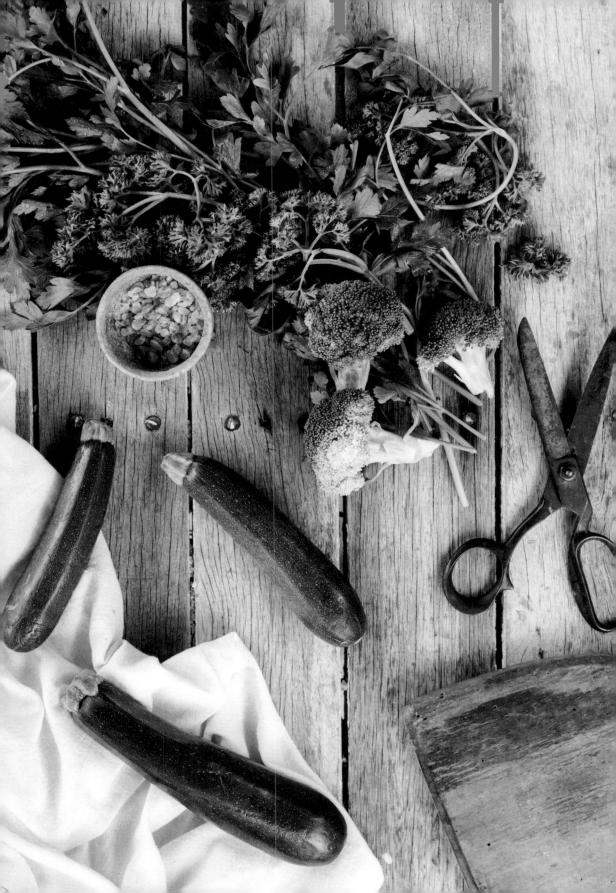

A rough guide to portion sizes is:

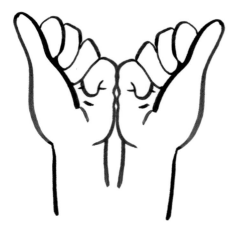

Two fist-sizes of concentrated food (like protein or carbohydrates), and then add as much non-starchy (high-water) vegetables as you like. If you have a high muscle mass or you are an athlete, you will likely need to adjust this.

Plan

Planning your weekly meals helps to reduce wasted food. If you shop to your plan, then everything in the fridge has a purpose, meaning heads of broccoli and bunches of spinach won't be forgotten and left to rot in the back of the fridge. By planning your meals, you will also reduce some of the perceived stress that can be involved in deciding what to have for dinner. You will even be less likely to reach for expensive takeaways when you have a plan in place.

Buy in bulk

Buying in bulk and sharing with a friend or storing for later use can be a great way to save money. Often when buying in bulk it is possible to get cheaper prices. Buying nuts and seeds in bulk can save you money long-term. Most nuts and seeds can be frozen to keep them fresh and stop them from going rancid. In-season produce can be frozen, bottled or fermented for later use.

Use your freezer

Freeze foods before they go to waste. Freezing brown bananas (peel them first), and saving them to be used in muffins or in a smoothie is a great way to reduce waste. The same can be done with other produce. Fruits can be stewed and then frozen, and later added to smoothies or warmed and added to muesli. Vegetable scraps can be saved and used to make stock or broth. Be sure to label food with what it is and the date on which you froze it, so that you don't end up with miscellaneous items in the freezer that never get used.

Grow your own

There are plenty of vegies and herbs that are easy to grow all year round. Kale, spinach and silverbeet will grow almost all year round, and can be used to make smoothies and juices, or to bulk out stews, curries, soups or salads. Herbs can be expensive to buy in small amounts, but they are very easy to grow. Parsley, thyme and rosemary are hardy herb plants, and so versatile, lending themselves to many dishes.

Explore your priorities

When it comes to what you spend your money on, consider your priorities. Do you draw the line at broccoli when it goes over a specific price, yet you buy yourself a coffee or two each day? Do you really need that twelfth pair of shoes, but you can't justify spending money on nuts? Sometimes finances for food are genuinely limited, while, for others, better health would be achieved if finances were reallocated.

Evolution

THE TIMELINE OF WOMEN

Science suggests that humans have been on the planet for about 150,000 years. Imagine that expanse of time as a 30-centimetre school ruler. If 30 centimetres represents 150,000 years, then 1 millimetre on that school ruler represents 500 years. Fast-forward to explore the last 100 years.

Consider what life was like for women in 1915. World War 1 had not long started. Twenty-five years later, in 1940, World War 2 had started, and this was really the first time that large numbers of women from across the social classes entered the workforce — not even 100 years ago. Skip forward another 25 years to 1965, which was not long after the media had announced to the world that an oral contraceptive pill was now available to women, which subsequently played a major role in shaping not only women's health, but women's participation in society and the choices available to them. Moving forward 25 more years to 1990, and the world has only just seen the end of the reign of its first female head of a global power, Margaret Thatcher… bringing us to today.

Now consider the past 10 to 20 years, and contemplate the rate of change we have asked our bodies to undergo due to all of the changes in our environment. Social media is only just over 10 years old. Remember when you left the house and no one could get hold of you until you returned home again?

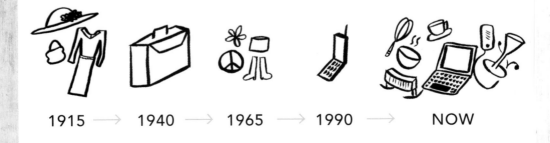

1915 ⟶ 1940 ⟶ 1965 ⟶ 1990 ⟶ NOW

Not to mention the changes in the food supply. Never ever before in the entirety of human history have we had access to so much refined sugar and starch, rancid fats, preservatives, artificial colours, flavours, sweeteners... The list goes on. Processed foods are still very new to our bodies. While there has always been change and stress hormone production, never before as a species have we undergone change at this rate, nor have we had the constant, relentless output of stress hormones. And this is creating some major health challenges today.

I frame this for you now in your *Women's Wellness Wisdom* journey, so that you can keep it in mind as you explore other aspects of your health. I want you to remember how new — how utterly foreign — so much that we experience today is to our body and our nervous system. Sure, we will evolve and adapt over time, but for now, for this generation and possibly a few more to come, our bodies are not at all used to much of what we throw at them — physically, nutritionally or emotionally.

So be kind to yourself and build a strong foundation for your physical and emotional wellbeing.

This means taking care of how you:
- eat
- drink
- move
- sleep
- think
- breathe
- believe, and
- perceive.

Let's create a way of life that best serves your physical, nutritional and emotional health.

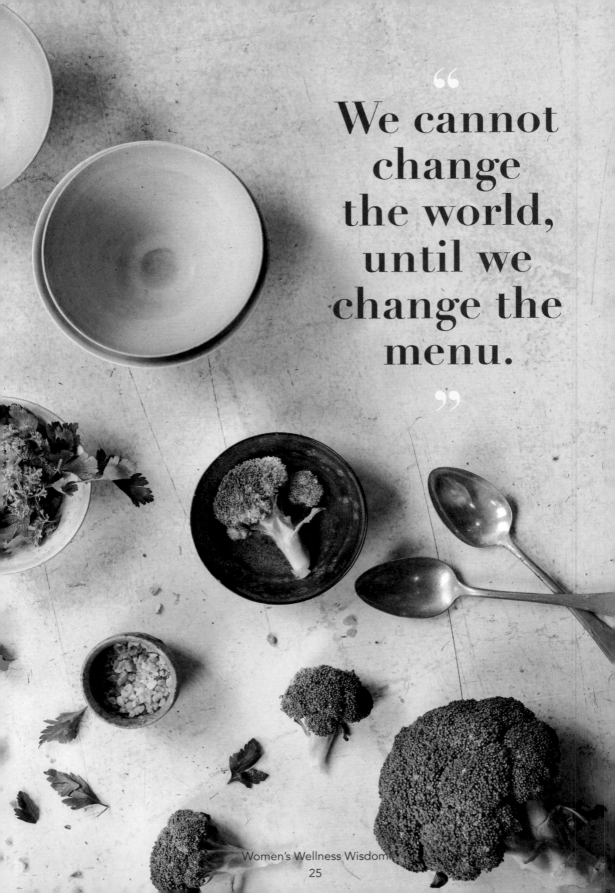

> " We cannot
> change
> the world,
> until we
> change the
> menu. "

It's up to you

TAKING RESPONSIBILITY FOR
YOUR NOURISHMENT

Some of the writing I do for newspapers and magazines involves answering readers' questions. These questions are mixed and varied, of course, but a couple of regular themes are: How am I supposed to eat well when I don't have time to cook? How can I look after my family when I just don't have the time to prepare meals from scratch?

Firstly, I do believe that, in general, we need to undergo a priority check and explore our values. While I appreciate that many of us are juggling many different tasks and roles daily, there is nothing on Earth that replaces the power of a nourishing diet. It is a basic foundational necessity of human life — well, certainly life with good-quality health.

Preparing real food may take more time, but it is time we have to allow for in our day. When we say "I don't have time" for something, what we are essentially saying is "that is not a priority for me". So try that on. How do you feel when you say to yourself that preparing a nourishing dinner is not a priority for you? The reality is we cannot compromise our nutrition and expect to still have fantastic health.

In saying all of that, though, there are a number of ways you can add nourishment to your meals that don't take much time. For example, chop up a mixture of greens, spinach, kale and herbs, and stir them through a stir-fry, salad, or soup — this is a great way to add a little nourishment-booster. Prepare big batches of meals on the weekend and freeze them for eating during the week, or stick to one-pot/pan meals packed full of vegetables. I cannot encourage you enough to explore how to make having a nourishing meal a priority for you.

You are worth taking care of.

Soil

THE BEGINNING OF WELLNESS...

From the soil, health and energy are born. The soil contains minerals which we need to live, such as calcium and magnesium. But we can't eat the soil, so we need a medium that is able to supply us with the Earth's nutrients. The middlemen are plants, as they absorb the nutrients from the soil and make them available to us as food. Isn't that an incredible way to think about how we obtain the nutrients that sustain our life?

However, if the soil is deficient in nutrients, then those nutrients are not in the food. So the quality of the soil where our food is grown plays an enormous role in how we feel, function and look each day.

Shop at local farmers' markets if they are available where you live. That way you can buy local produce, get to know your farmers, find out how they tend to the food you buy, and you can thank them for their hard work. Without their care and efforts, it is impossible for us to have great health. It seems crazy to me that most people know the name of their doctor but not the names of their farmers.

Decreasing soil quality, the nutritional demands of increased stress hormone production, as well as our exposure (via air, skin, food and drinks) to more and more problematic substances requiring detoxification, are all reasons that have contributed to me designing a range of plant-based nutritional supports derived purely from foods. The bioavailability of nutrients from foods is considered to be superior to those that are synthetically created and they offer you a helping hand when it comes to optimal nourishment.

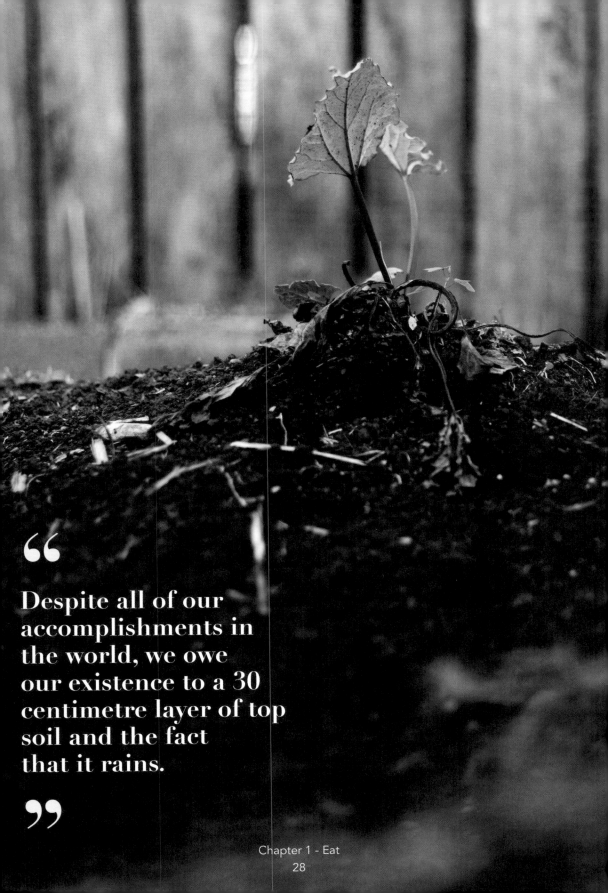

> " Despite all of our
> accomplishments in
> the world, we owe
> our existence to a 30
> centimetre layer of top
> soil and the fact
> that it rains. "

Nature

WHY NATURE GETS IT RIGHT AND
HUMAN INTERVENTION GETS IT WRONG

Inside your digestive system, you have all of the equipment (digestive enzymes, for example) with which to break down and extract the energy and the nutrients from the food you eat. Your food is the only way your body obtains energy for you to use and experience. Why would you want to interfere with that? Think about it. When you are tired, everything is more difficult. It impacts on the food that you choose, whether you get off the couch and go for a walk or not, the jobs that you would apply for, the friends that you make, your self-talk and the way you speak to the people you love the most in this world.

When it comes to food, Nature gets it right and human intervention can unfortunately get it so wrong. Researchers in the United States have developed a camera that is the size of a vitamin capsule that you can swallow, and it allows 15 hours of footage to be shot from inside the digestive system. This totally spins my tyres. The researchers gave one group of people a real-food meal made of noodles, which they had made from scratch from flour and water, and then served in a broth, which had been made from vegetables, water and salt. The other group were given a meal of noodles bought from the supermarket, and which contained 15 different ingredients. These noodles were served with a broth, which was made of water added to the sachet of powder that came with the noodles. This bought-food meal was served with a blue-coloured drink. Both groups ate their meals and then swallowed the cameras.

Four hours later, all that was left in the digestive tracts of those who had eaten the homemade, real-food was white fluff. Everything was well broken down, the way it is supposed to be. For the bought-food group, four hours after eating and

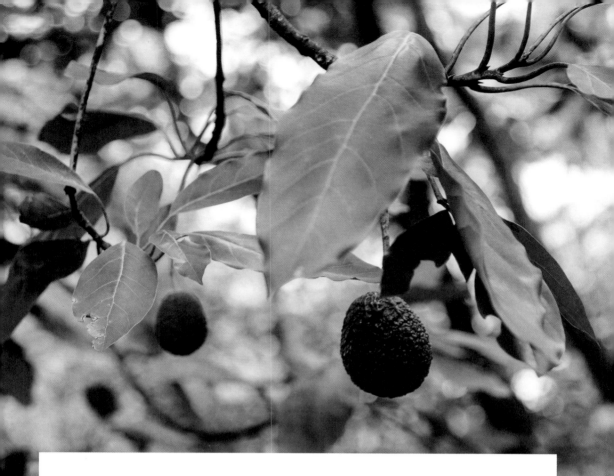

swallowing the camera, you could still see the teeth marks in the noodles. When you have had "food" exposed to your digestive system's equipment for four hours, and it is still relatively intact, this suggests that this "food" may contain substances which we have no capacity to break down. Remember, food is the only way we obtain physical energy. Plus, on top of this, the noodles in the bought-food group had turned blue from the blue drink. This was because the dye was petroleum-based, and we have nothing inside of us that allows us to break down petrol. This may sound ludicrous to you, but this is our reality. We think that, because something is on a shelf for us to buy, it must be okay. But there are no guarantees that it is.

So when it comes to food, choose low human intervention (HI) food. Choose real-food. Wholefood. This is food after all. There is no such thing as "junk food". There is only "junk" or there is "food".

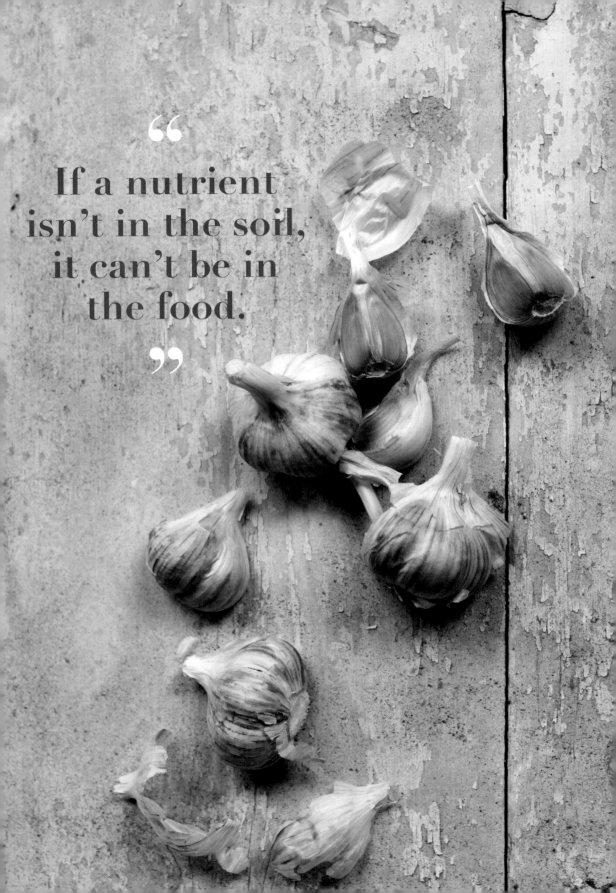

> **If a nutrient isn't in the soil, it can't be in the food.**

Supplements

THE POWER OF PLANTS AS FOOD AND SUPPLEMENTS

There are many reasons I am a fan of nutritional supplementation — although not all supplements are created equally. In other words, they don't all impact on the body in the same the way. The quality and the source of the nutrients, as well as what else they are packaged with, all play a role in their bioavailability (usability) for your body.

Here are a few reasons why I like good-quality nutritional supplementation:

- If a nutrient isn't in the soil, it can't be in our food. Too much food today is significantly lower in nutrients than it was even 50 years ago.

- We are exposed to more pollutants today, via what we eat, drink, breathe, and put on our skin. Pollutants require detoxification: biochemical pathways that change problematic substances into less harmful versions of themselves. These processes require nutrients, meaning we need more nutrients today, not fewer. So much of our health, energy and disease prevention is related to detoxification and elimination, and nutrients are required for these processes to work effectively.

- When we make stress hormones, it changes how we breathe to being more rapid and shallow breaths. This turns over more oxygen, which means that more free radicals are generated. These free radicals have the potential to damage our tissues in a process called oxidative damage, one of the ways we age and degenerate from the inside out. (Note that we also make free radicals during detoxification, so the more pollutants we are exposed to, the more free radicals we will generate as well.) To combat the effects of more free radicals, we must consume antioxidants to nullify their effect.

Antioxidants are found primarily in coloured plant foods. Yet here is another big change that has occurred in the recent past: the antioxidant levels in our foods have dropped dramatically. Why? Well, while plants have the ability to protect themselves from pests by making certain substances within themselves, if the plant is sprayed to protect it from pests, it doesn't produce these innate protective substances. It has no need. And many of these substances that would naturally protect the plant — but that are now not being made by the plant, due to spraying — are antioxidants to humans when we consume them. Hence their decreased availability to us.

I am also a fan of getting as much nutrition as possible from our food, particularly plants. Plants are little superstars when it comes to what they are able to do for us. Consider the Brassica genus of vegetables, for example. They contain not only vitamins, minerals and fibre, but also substances unique to this botanical family — substances known as indoles and glucoraphanin, which gets converted into the ultra-superstar sulphoraphane. These substances support the optimal functioning of some of our most important biochemical pathways: those of the liver, and particularly those needed for essential estrogen and pesticide detoxification.

Then there is beetroot. This stunningly-coloured plant contains many nutritious substances, including nitrates which convert to nitric oxide. This can help regulate blood pressure and provide better oxygen delivery to the tissues — again, essential for great energy, anti-aging and disease prevention.

Blackcurrants (with their seeds in), grapes (with their seeds in) and berries are also superstars with their oligomeric proanthocyanidins (OPCs), which are a set of bioflavonoid complexes that act as free radical scavengers in the human body. Many names refer to this set of bioflavonoids, including leuco-anthocyanin, anthocyanidin and many more. Think of OPCs as being nutrients with super-powers: they support virtually every metabolic system in the body. Research has shown that decent intakes of OPCs help protect against cardiovascular and other degenerative diseases, and have numerous other benefits, including lowering LDL cholesterol levels, reducing platelet aggregation (you don't want your blood to be too sticky for so many reasons), increasing the strength and elasticity of blood vessels, helping collagen repair itself, reducing fluid retention and inflammation, relieving functional problems associated with varicose veins, lessening the tendency toward diabetic retinopathy, and improving skin health. All of that from Nature.

This shows the power inherent in our food. Yet remember that the nutrient density in our food is completely reliant on soil health. And the usability of nutrients by the body can also be impacted on based on their source.

For example, did you know that most nutritional supplements are synthetic, and are made in a laboratory? Arguably, vitamin C is vitamin C no matter what. Certainly, vitamin C is ascorbic acid, and ascorbic acid can be created in a laboratory or by Nature in, for example, an orange or a lemon. Both sources behave as vitamin C in the body. Yet studies have been undertaken to examine the effectiveness of a number of nutrients based on their source: synthetically produced or as nutrients from food. The food source wins almost every time.

It seems, then, that there are compounds unique to food that make nutrients highly bioavailable. So in a world where soil is depleted and our nutritional needs are greater than ever before, I have seen great health be obtained and maintained through eating well, and supplementing this with additional nutrients and herbs from wholefood, real-food and plant sources.

Could the way you eat do with a nutritional boost?

How are you going to do this?

Check out *www.drlibby.com* for more information on my personal range of products to assist your health.

Healing herbs
MEDICINAL PROPERTIES OF PLANTS

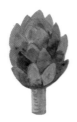

Globe artichoke
(Cynara scolymus)

- Supports bile production from the liver, crucial for detoxifying estrogen, pesticides and other fat-soluble substances

- Stimulates lymphatic flow

- Great for sex hormone balance, particularly if estrogen is in excess.

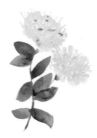

Rhodiola
(Rhodiola roseaw)

- Lowers cortisol

- Improves lowered mood

- Improves energy

- Improves the body's response to stress (which can have an exceptional ripple effect on all of the body systems negatively affected by stress).

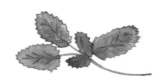

Lemon balm
(Melissa officinalis)

- Helps to decrease nervous agitation

- Soothes and calms the digestive system if stress is playing a role in the discomfort (bloating, flatulence, colic)

- Supports good-quality sleep.

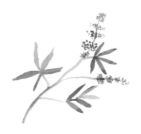

Chaste tree
(Vitex agnus-castus)

- Fosters communication between the pituitary gland and the ovaries to help support regular ovulation

- Helps support a regular menstrual cycle.

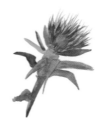

St Mary's thistle
(Silybum marianum)

- Stimulates liver detoxification
- Stimulates lymphatic flow
- Helps damaged liver cells regenerate
- Helps protect liver cells from alcohol and other hepatotoxins.

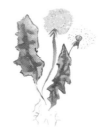

Dandelion leaf and root
(Taraxacum officinale)

- The leaves act as a diuretic, supporting healthy fluid balance, and can help relieve fluid retention

- The root stimulates liver detoxification and lymphatic flow.

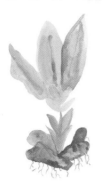

Turmeric
(Curcuma longa)

- Powerful anti-inflammatory

- Supports liver detoxification

- An excellent antioxidant (mops up free radicals, which can cause aging and degeneration from the inside out)

- Supports a healthy immune system.

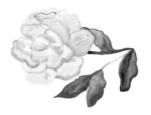

Peony
(Paeonia lactiflora)

- Great for period pain (dysmenorrhoea), as it relaxes smooth muscle, is an analgesic and is an anti-spasmodic herb

- Helps support pain relief in premenstrual tension, endometriosis, polycystic ovarian syndrome and fibroids

- Helps re-establish a healthy sex hormone balance.

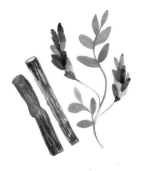

Licorice
(Glycyrrhiza glabra)

- Adrenal restorative herb critical to healthy cortisol levels

- Helps healthy energy production

- Improves progesterone production due to better adrenal function

- Teams up amazingly with paeonia to relieve painful menstruation.

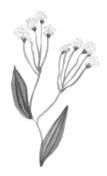

Bupleurum
(Bupleurum falcatum)

- Stimulates liver detoxification

- Indicated if clots in menstrual blood.

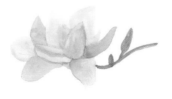

Magnolia
(Magnolia officinalis)

- Helps to decrease anxious feelings

- Helps to relieve nervous tension

- Supports good-quality sleep.

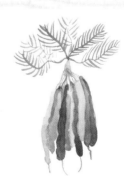

Shatavari
(Asparagus racemosus)

- Reproductive system tonic from menses to menopause

- Supports fertility

- Calming to the nervous system.

Food language

FOOD IS NOT "HEALTHY"

Have you ever thought about the language you have adopted when it comes to describing food? I don't mean its flavours and the latest hot-spots to eat, but rather the traits of the food itself. This applies particularly around the use of the word "healthy" — which I have seen used to describe everything from kale to low-fat processed foods. It is time we became more accurate in our use of language about food, not just for ourselves, but because it impacts on the way we teach children, which in turn will impact on the way they relate to food and to the choices they will make across their lifetimes.

Foods aren't healthy — they are nutritious. Or not. Humans are healthy. Or we are not. Instead of describing foods as "healthy" or "unhealthy", it is more accurate and more beneficial to consider whether they are nutritious or nourishing. With the popularity of the low-fat era, and to a certain extent because of dieting language, it has been easy for too many people to consider food as nothing more than the calories (a measure of energy) that it supplies. Yet, obviously food is so much more than that: the food you eat literally becomes a part of you, and it is the vitamins and minerals in nutritious foods that keep us alive. Really think about that.

The concept of whether or not a food is good for us has become far too confusing as we have more and more, often-conflicting but well-meaning, voices in the health and nutrition world. A great way to strip nutrition or health information back and make sense of it all is to bring it back to the fundamentals of good health, which most health professionals, regardless of their background, agree on. These include: eat more vegetables; decrease or omit refined sugars; avoid or minimize processed meats; stay hydrated; base meals and snacks on real, wholefoods; sleep well; sit less; move more; and maintain (or preferably build) muscle mass.

I think it is also incredibly important to remember that, while there are some core nutrition fundamentals that benefit most people, there is no one-size-fits-all when it comes to how we nourish our bodies. Your body is your best barometer — notice how certain foods make you feel and pay attention to any patterns. Food is supposed to energize you; if what you are eating is consistently making you tired, it may not be serving your health. Remember that the parts of your body that sadden or frustrate you are simply messengers asking you to eat, drink, move, think, breathe, believe or perceive in a new way. See them as the gifts that they are. Your own body knows what is best for it.

> **Make NUTRITIOUS food choices to support your HEALTH.**

Children

TEACH CHILDREN THE NUTRITIONAL VALUE OF FOOD

We all want our little humans to be well-nourished — body, mind and soul. And whole, real-food is the best food for them (and us). Teaching children from the get-go about the nutritional value of food can be game-changing for their future choices, as well as for their health right now. Instead of suggesting that they eat something because it is "healthy" (a word that has no connotation to most three-year-olds), explain, for example, that an orange is a good food choice because it contains vitamin C, and this helps your body to not catch a cold. Even from a young age, when children start to hear the "so what" — the reason the orange is a good choice for them — they are more likely to eat the food.

The flip-side is also true. Given that it is nutrients that keep us alive, and most processed foods are very low in nutrients (with some even containing substances that can take away from good health and energy), then processed foods are not wise everyday choices. When you base your explanations to children about food on nourishment (what the food contains and why this helps them), then you can explain that a highly processed food doesn't contain anything that helps them, and so it is best that they only eat these foods at birthday parties (irregularly). It is, after all, what we do every day that impacts on our health, not what we do occasionally.

Currently, in developed countries there are 42 million obese children between the ages of zero and five years. If this trajectory continues, by 2025 there will be 70 million obese children. As adults, we are 100 per cent responsible for that. That statement is not designed to elicit guilt. It is just how it is. Children are too young to make their own food choices at that age. We need to be their guides; and they also watch what we do. But take a moment to also consider what happens for those zero- to five-year-olds who are currently obese. Studies show that they are more likely to become obese teenagers if they are obese when they are very young. More body fat means more estrogen production for boys and girls, as the larger the number and the larger the size of the body fat cells, the more estrogen will be produced, and at younger and younger ages. This is already having dire consequences the world over, with girls not yet at double-digit ages being able to give birth, given that more estrogen tends to promote the earlier onset of menstruation (menarche).

The older children become, the more they will have created their own perception about what is "healthy". For some children "healthy" and "food" in the same sentence is a win and something they want to partake in. While for others, they link "healthy" to "yuck". Use the information in "Food is not 'healthy'" to help you shift your language patterns about food, and pass this on to your children. Help them, through food language and nourishing explanations, to primarily make nutritious food choices, by explaining how nutritious foods help them. Link nutritious food choices to what they care about (for example, being a good rugby player or being strong), rather than to your focus.

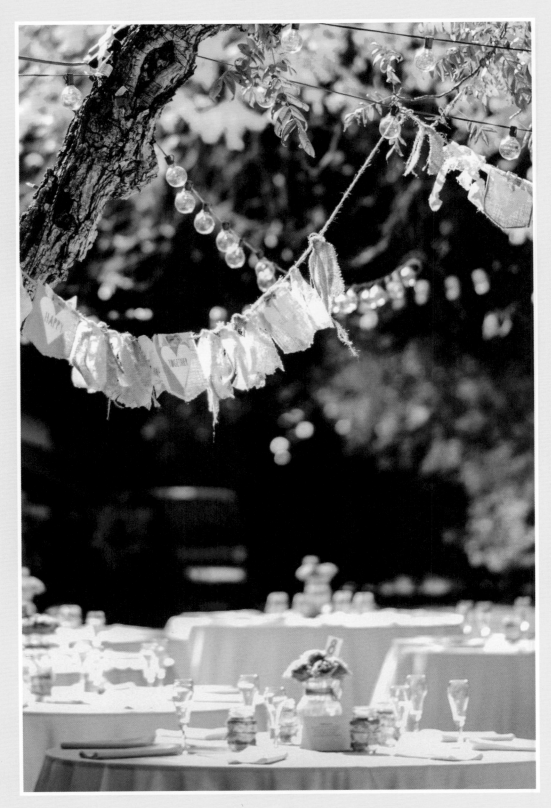

Women's Wellness Wisdom

How to eat

BE A "FLEXITARIAN" WHEN IT COMES TO YOUR HEALTH AND FOOD CHOICES

Have you noticed that every possible way of eating has a name now? More and more people are labelling the way they eat, and judging others who have a different idea of health and wellness to their own. While it's fantastic to see more people taking an active interest in their wellbeing, these labels often come with strict rules. Such sets of criteria around what is acceptable and what is not may work for some, but for others it just simply isn't sustainable.

To ease the situation, I came up with the term "Flexitarian" to describe how I eat, as the term best suits my philosophy. It is about listening to what will best serve your body, health, energy (note: this does not mean tastebuds rule the choice!), and even your spiritual practice. Sometimes if we run our food choices by a label someone else has told us to follow, we can miss the messages of our body's needs.

The concept of being a "Flexitarian" can be used by anyone, and it simply means you don't have stringent rules. You might instead prefer to approach how you nourish yourself with the idea that you have high standards. In other words, you don't choose that highly-processed, sugar- and preservative-laden snack because someone told you not to. You don't eat it because it doesn't serve your health, quality of life or your longevity. You don't eat it because you care about yourself. That's great! But, having said that, please always remember that it is what you do every day that impacts on your health, not what you do occasionally. Feeling guilty about the odd poor-quality food choice does nothing for your health, either.

If you are someone who is energized and uplifted by strict rules, or if you have an illness that requires you to eat exceptionally at all times, then please continue to do that. You know if this is you. If you are someone, however, who fears food or weight gain, or uses food as a mechanism of control in your life, then you might want to consider relaxing a little. Rigidity when it stems from fear does not serve our health in any way.

A gentler approach can embrace a degree of flexibility, or what some like to call "zig and zag".

A "zig" meal is made up of nutrient-dense foods, real-foods and no alcohol, whereas for a "zag" meal, the focus is more about the company you are in, being playful and relaxing. Zags are part of a healthy and sustainable lifestyle. If this approach is going to serve someone's health, I would guide someone to zag once a week, or for three out of their 35 eating occasions. (If you eat three meals and two snacks each day, this is 35 eating occasions. Some of you will eat more frequently than that, some of you less frequently — I have taken 35 as a weekly average.) For others, five zag occasions better suits them. That's still 30 meals that are of a nutritionally high quality.

If you know you are going to your office party, or to a friend's birthday, that doesn't mean the whole day is a write-off, yet so many people approach their life or health in this way. Having the office party in the evening is even more reason to eat a nutritious breakfast and lunch, following up with nutrient-dense food choices the next day.

You enjoy the zag, but, when you live mostly as a zig, the zag takes very little toll on your overall level of wellbeing.

The "Flexitarian" concept can also apply to your choice of movement. It simply means that you make a conscious effort to move regularly, but if you don't your whole world won't collapse and you won't suddenly gain four kilograms.

When we are kinder to ourselves and put less pressure on fulfilling set criteria, we are more likely to make choices in our lives that we can sustain.

After all, the way you take care of yourself needs to be sustainable.

How you need to eat for your best nourishment often changes over time. I want to encourage you to be in touch with what your body wants and provide it with the nourishment it needs. When it comes to your food choices, if you need a name for how you eat, call it "Just Eat Real Food" or "Flexitarian", meaning you are flexible to the needs of your body (this does not mean your taste buds) as they change over time; or be a "Qualitarian", choosing good-quality whole, real-food.

ZIG

NUTRIENT-DENSE FOODS, REAL-FOODS AND NO ALCOHOL

ZAG

THE FOCUS IS MORE ABOUT THE COMPANY YOU ARE IN, BEING PLAYFUL AND RELAXING

Cut it out?

HOW DO YOU KNOW IF YOU NEED TO BE GLUTEN FREE OR DAIRY FREE – OR BOTH?

Refined sugars don't serve anyone's health. If you haven't done so already, get them really low or omit them from how you eat. It's easy and it's essential to every body system inside you. There are tips on how to do this throughout this book, as I know many of you will have scoffed at the "it's easy" comment above.

It can seriously though, just be a decision that you care enough about yourself that the white stuff – that doesn't contain any nutrition does not belong in your body. In this moment, we could all raise our standards when it comes to what we eat and drink. And for some, it's that simple. If it's not that easy for you though, explore the strategies offered throughout this book to get your refined sugars to low or zero.

But what about being gluten free? Or dairy free? Is this necessary? Having worked with people one-on-one for over two decades, following are the clues that I use to guide me to guide you.

Considering these guidelines, is there a dietary trial you are keen to undertake to see how you feel and what symptoms may resolve as a result?

You need to keep in mind that the trial is four to eight weeks out of your very long life that may offer you great insight into your health, or not. If you continue with this way of eating beyond eight weeks, it is essential that you consult an experienced health professional to ensure you are meeting your nutritional requirements.

CONSIDER...

FOUR TO EIGHT WEEK DIETARY TRIALS

Trial a gluten-free way of eating if you have:

- An autoimmune disease or elevated autoantibodies
- A strong Irish heritage
- Gut-based symptoms or a gut-central disease
- Unexplained fatigue, dry skin, hair and nails and a tendency to constipation

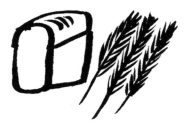

Trial a dairy-free way of eating if you have:

- Have a history of recurrent (or current) streptococcus-based infections such as tonsillitis, ear infections, chest infections, bronchitis
- Have a history of (or current) eczema
- Have chronic sinus problems
- Clear your throat constantly
- Have recurring excessive flatulence with an offensive odour
- Mostly breathe through your mouth

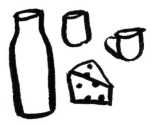

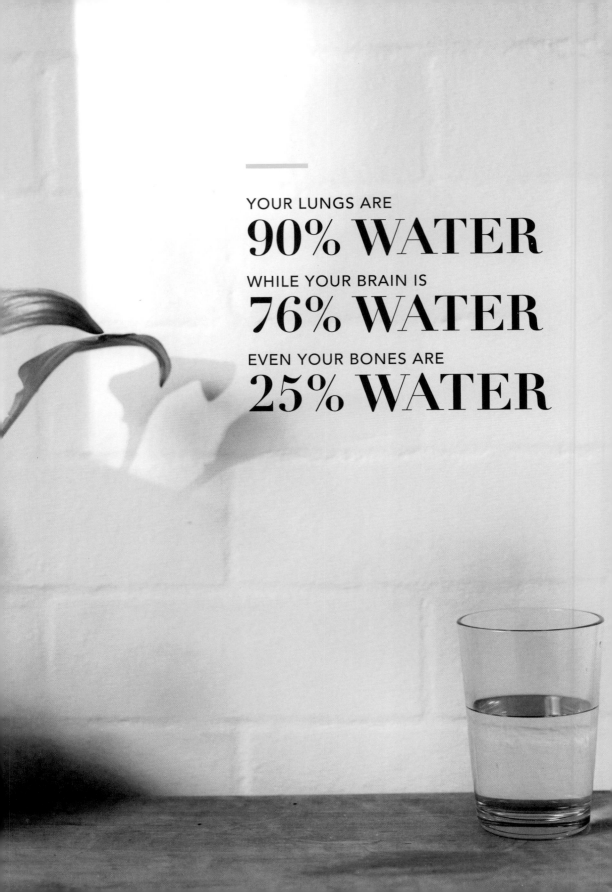

YOUR LUNGS ARE
90% WATER
WHILE YOUR BRAIN IS
76% WATER
EVEN YOUR BONES ARE
25% WATER

Hydration

WHY WATER NEEDS TO BE YOUR MAIN DRINK

Water is the basis of all life, and that includes your body. The muscles that move your body are 75 per cent water. Your blood, which is responsible for transporting nutrients throughout your body, is 82 per cent water. Your lungs, which take oxygen from the air, are 90 per cent water, while your brain is 76 per cent water. Even your bones are 25 per cent water!

Great hydration is essential for health, and of course the skin loves it. But the skin is simply a reflection of interior processes. Scientists believe that when we are born we are about 75 per cent water, but by the time we are 30 most adults' total body water content has dropped to around 57–60 per cent. Few people do well to maintain 70 per cent. Think about this. Somewhere between about 57 and 70 per cent of your physical body is water. Wow. No wonder the impact of dehydration is significant on our inner health and outer sparkle.

Our health is truly dependent on the quality and quantity of the water we drink. Unintentional chronic dehydration can contribute to pain and inflammation in the body, and it can even be involved in the development of many degenerative diseases. Helping your body prevent such ills by ensuring great-quality water intake on a regular basis is a crucial step with any lifestyle plan.

Following is an article I wrote for a magazine, which contains plenty of useful information to help better support your hydration efforts.

THE WONDER OF WATER:
THE KEY TO HAPPY, HEALTHY CELLS

When it comes to water, most people believe they need to drink more than they currently do, and, without a conscious effort, this never seems to happen. The wonders of water are well-documented, ranging from fostering glowing, clear skin and eyes to the prevention of kidney stones. Yet, as with most nutritional information, there is conflicting information out there, which makes it difficult for individuals to truly know how much is enough.

The science

Without water, a human will usually only live for a mere three days. So essential is this liquid to our survival that we need it more than food. Science currently tells us that we need 33 millilitres (mL) of water for each kilogram (kg) of our body weight. A 70-kilogram person, therefore, requires 2,310 millilitres (2.31 litres) a day. However, we tend to forget that many plant foods have a high water content, and this contributes to our overall daily water consumption. Herbal teas and soups also add up. Foods and drinks containing caffeine and alcohol, however, draw water out of our body, so the larger their presence in our diet, the greater our fluid requirements.

Fruits and vegetables are almost always over 70 per cent water, so the more of these we eat, the less we need to consume as fluid. Naturally, perspiration and increased breathing rates generated by exercise and/or stress increase our need for water, but the specific amounts necessary are difficult to determine and will be highly individual. Trust your thirst when it comes to this. Thirst is Nature's way of letting you know you need to drink!

Thirst and hydration

Some people rarely feel thirsty, while for others their thirst never seems quenched. Some people resist increasing their fluid intake as they tire of frequently running to the loo. Yet, for others, increasing their fluid intake makes them feel swollen and uncomfortable. With all of these different scenarios, it is not surprising that there is so much conflicting information out there. So what's behind these differences, and what can you do about it?

Just because you drink water, or even enough water for adequate hydration, does not necessarily mean that the cells of your body are hydrated. Ideally, every cell of your body looks like a grape; this is the case when your cells are hydrated. A dehydrated state means your cells appear more like raisins and this can be the result of inadequate water intake, a lack of minerals, or poor adrenal gland function, often due to chronic stress, physical and/ or emotional trauma, or excess caffeine or alcohol consumption.

To absorb the water you drink into your cells, you need calcium, magnesium, sodium, potassium and chloride. Some of these minerals make their home inside the cell, while others reside outside the cell wall. These minerals all talk to each other, and if one is present at an excessively high level or, alternatively, if one of those minerals is lacking, it can be difficult for water to enter the cell. Physically, when water stays outside the cell, it manifests as a feeling of fluid retention, which for some people is so noticeable that clothing will cut into them as the day progresses. You can begin to change this by improving the mineral balance of your diet and taking care of your liver.

One of the best ways to improve your mineral intake and balance is to base your diet on what I have come to call low "human intervention" (HI) food. Most plant foods get their minerals from the soil in which they are grown, so foods that come from organic, biodynamic, or permacultured soils tend to be superior in their mineral profile. Green leafy vegies have a broad mineral profile that includes calcium, magnesium and potassium. Nuts and seeds also pack a powerful mineral punch, and make a great snack or addition to any meal.

Minerals

People with low blood pressure often feel better with a slightly reduced fluid intake, as excess water may dilute their blood levels of minerals. Increasing your intake of all of the minerals above can, however, make a significant difference in that low blood pressure feeling and experience.

Your body uses minerals to, among other things, create electrolytes. Often described as the "sparks of life", electrolytes carry electrical currents through the body, sending instructions to cells in all body systems. Electrolytes are also necessary for enzyme production. Enzymes are responsible for the biochemical processes that drive the function of the body, as well as for digesting food and absorbing nutrients, and they impact on muscle function as well as hormone production. Poor mineral intake and/or balance, as well as dehydration, therefore, affect all body systems and functions.

Amp up your mineral intake

A healthy and balanced way to increase the amount of minerals in your diet is to amp up the amount of plant foods you currently consume, the green-coloured ones in particular. Add them wherever you can, and do your best to base your evening meal on greens, rather than their being a token effort on the side of the plate. You can also include Celtic sea salt or Himalayan pink salt. They typically contain 84 minerals that can help your body better absorb water into the cells. Adding good-quality salt to your food can be of particular importance if you eat limited or no processed foods, particularly if you suffer with digestive system problems or low blood pressure. Be sure that iodine is one of the trace minerals in the salt that you use.

Juicing or blending fruits and vegetables is also a great way to increase the fluid and mineral content of your diet and ensure that water is absorbed into your cells. If fluid retention is an ongoing challenge for you, try juicing celery, cucumber, mint and a small amount of pineapple daily for a week. Supplementing with a "green drink" powder can also be highly beneficial.

Set up rituals in your day to flag your memory that it is time to drink. Start your day with a glass of warm water with lemon juice, for example. Make drinking enough pure water a habit in your life. It won't take long for you to feel the benefits. Water is a simple and wonderful investment in your long-term health.

SIGNS

DEHYDRATED	HYDRATED
Shrivelled and dry skin that lacks elasticity and doesn't "bounce back" when pinched into a fold	Plump, "bounce back" when pinched into a fold (skin)
Sunken eyes	Fine lines less pronounced (skin)
A feeling of tightness or tautness (skin)	Less or no feeling of tightness or tautness (skin)
Fine lines emphasized (skin)	A look or feeling of softness
Lack of concentration	Bright, clear eyes
Feelings of dizziness	Strong hair and nails
Bad breath (dehydration can decrease saliva production)	Tears form easily when crying
Dry, sticky mouth	Alertness/less tiredness
Irritability	
Headaches	
Constipation	
Minimal urine	
Muscle cramps	
Few tears when crying	

Caffeine

WHAT HAPPENS WHEN YOU CONSUME CAFFEINE?

Over 90 per cent of adults in the Western world consume caffeine daily. More than 50 per cent of Americans consume 13 or more caffeinated drinks per week. In Australia and New Zealand, studies suggest that caffeine consumption has more than tripled since the 1960s, and, although levels may not be on par with rates of consumption in the United States, they are rapidly rising, not only due to an increase in coffee consumption, but also due to the widespread use of caffeine as an ingredient in, for example, energy drinks.

In the United States, 70 per cent of soft drinks contain caffeine. In a US study conducted in 2011, 28 per cent of coffee drinkers had their first cup within 15 minutes of waking and 68 per cent within an hour of waking, while 57 per cent added sugar or sweetener to their brew. The level of caffeine consumption for far too many people is considered addictive by medical textbook standards.

Here's what happens when you consume caffeine. Caffeine sends a message to the pituitary gland in your brain that it needs to send a message to the adrenal glands to make stress hormones: adrenalin and/or cortisol. When adrenalin is released, your blood sugar elevates to provide you with more energy (fuel) to escape from the danger that the stress hormones communicate you are in; your blood pressure and pulse rate rise to provide more oxygen to the muscles, which tense in preparation for action. Reproductive functions are down-regulated since they use a lot of energy and are not necessary for your immediate survival, given the impending "threat". Plus, your body does not believe it is safe to bring a baby into what it perceives to be an unsafe world, as adrenalin tells your body that your life is in danger, and cortisol communicates that there is no more food left in the world!

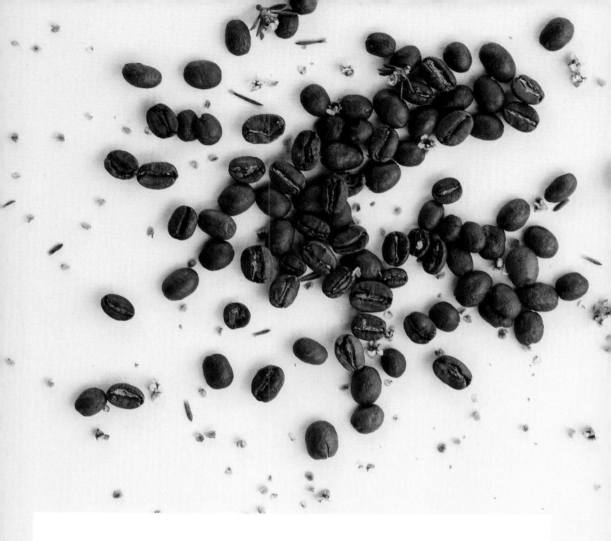

Adrenalin production can be the result of real or perceived stress, or simply the result of your caffeine intake. Caffeine, via the stress hormones, and coupled with the signal to activate the fight-or-flight response, fires you up. Once triggered, in this state you have little hope of being calm, centred and able to focus on any instructions being given to you; for example, by your boss, a colleague, or a receptionist confirming an appointment with you. In addition, this biochemical state puts all of its resources into saving your life rather than into what are considered non-vital processes, those inside you that nourish your skin, hair, nails and allow the reproductive system to work optimally. Over time, the lack of resources, such as nutrients, available to these so-called non-vital processes has significant consequences internally and externally. First, your skin, hair and nails won't receive the nutrients and other substances they need to look their best. Secondly, because the fuel that drives the fight-or-flight response is glucose ("sugar"), you will crave sugar to constantly refill your fuel tank, and you won't utilize your fat stores as often or as easily. Also, with additional glucose in your blood, you will release insulin — a fat-storage hormone — and it will first convert unused glucose from your blood into glycogen and store it in your muscles; what is left over is converted into body fat.

I am not suggesting you stop drinking caffeine — unless, that is, you fiercely want to hang onto it! What we resist is often what we need. Only you know if you are having too much. Many women would certainly benefit from taking a break from it for two menstrual cycles, though, while others would do well to reduce their intake to one caffeinated drink per day. If you are a genuinely chilled-out person, then caffeine probably just helps you focus, while too many people today have a low (or high) level of anxious feelings, and these are driven primarily by adrenalin — the very hormone that caffeine leads your body to release.

Following is a list of some common sources of caffeine.

Keep in mind that many cafés serve a double shot in their coffees, and that standard medical textbooks list "caffeine intoxication" as occurring with over 400 milligrams of caffeine consumed within eight hours.

Notice whether you feel calmer drinking weak black tea or green tea, because, although they contain caffeine, they also contain another substance called "theanine", which helps to buffer the effect of the caffeine, and this tends to lead to an alert but calm state.

We are all different in our tolerance of caffeine. I simply want you to be aware of yours. It may serve you best to have it only three times a week, instead of three a day. Or try one a day if you are used to more. Or take the plunge and take a break, particularly if you have premenstrual tension or pain with your menstrual cycle.

Common sources of caffeine

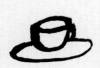

ESPRESSO
107 mg/serve

CAFE LATTE
(250ML)
113-282 mg/serve

INSTANT
COFFEE (250ML)
60-80 mg/serve

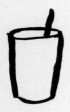

ICED COFFEE
(500ML)
30-200 mg/serve

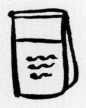

BREWED COFFEE
VENTI (600ML)
415 mg/serve

TEA
(250ML)
25-110 mg/serve

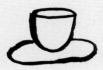

GREEN TEA
(250ML)
30-50 mg/serve

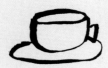

DECAF
(250ML)
2-5 mg/serve

COLA
(355ML)
36-48 mg/serve

ENERGY
DRINK (250ML)
80 mg/serve

DARK
CHOCOLATE (30G)
20 mg/serve

What's your plan with caffeine?

Alcohol

DOES IT LIGHT YOU UP OR DULL YOUR SHINE?

There is much insight to be gained even by how you approach this topic. If you are dreading it, there may be some behaviours that need to change.

Many people knowingly or unknowingly consume too much alcohol, and the effects of too much may silently or loudly reverberate through your life, not to mention the lives of those around you. An excess of alcohol can have traumatic effects in people's lives, or drive some major or minor health concerns. Whether it is increased body fat or cellulite, less energy and vitality, worse bouts of premenstrual syndrome or mood fluctuations... Or perhaps your get up and go has got up and left. As fun as it can be at the time, alcohol can rob you of your clarity and purpose. Too much, or consumed too often, it can take the edge off your vitality and your greatness.

Or it might be different times of the year that herald big statements about alcohol: January, after the Christmas parties and as part of a New Year's resolution; February, because it has the least number of days; Dry July or Oct-sober. Or it may be health challenges forcing us to make changes. I remember a famous person once intimating "never drink so much that you are diagnosed with an illness and then you can never drink again".

People drink for wide and varied reasons. For some, it is the way they socialize, or the way they wind down from the day. Some use alcohol to distract themselves from thoughts and feelings they would rather avoid. It can be a way that people cope. Regardless of the reason, many of us over-drink without even realizing it.

A standard drink is 10 grams of alcohol in whatever form that

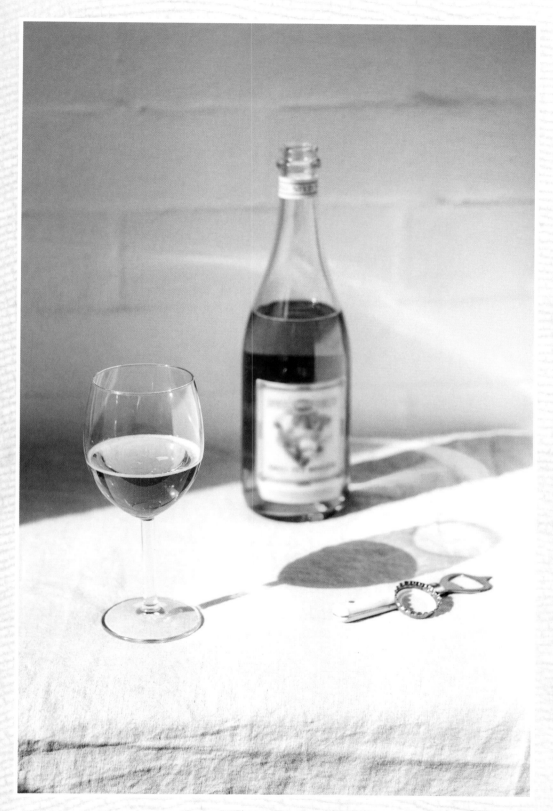

comes. In Australia and New Zealand, 10 grams of alcohol is a 330-millilitre bottle of 4 per cent beer, a 30-millilitre nip of spirits, 170-millilitre of champagne, and a measly 100-millilitre of wine — about four swallows! Next time you pour yourself a glass of wine, measure it and see what your natural pour is. For most, it is considerably more than 100-millilitres, and, as a result, many are over-drinking unknowingly.

The current recommendations provided by heart organizations say that for women no more than two standard drinks per day with two alcohol-free days per week is okay, while for men three standard drinks per day and two alcohol-free days is acceptable.

We have long heard the heart-health benefits of red wine publicly sung, and somehow it justifies to too many that drinking is okay — you tell yourself you are clearly looking after your heart. Also consider the World Cancer Research Fund's (WCRF) position statement on alcohol. They suggest that women have "less than one standard drink per day". They have found this to be even more important if you have a family history of cancer.

I'm not suggesting that you don't drink alcohol, if you like it. Alcohol consumption can be immensely pleasurable for those who partake. I simply want to appeal to you to get honest with yourself about how alcohol affects you. In your heart you know if you drink too much and when it is impacting negatively on your health. Alcohol can affect the way we relate to those we love the most in the world, and of course it affects how we feel about ourselves. It has a depressant action on the human nervous system, so anyone who often experiences low moods is best served avoiding it, or certainly only consuming it on very special occasions. If you drink, drink for the pleasure of it, rather than the misconstrued message that alcohol is good for your health.

The link between the consistent over-consumption of alcohol and breast cancer is undeniable. Research has shown this time and time again, and for many years now. Yet we rarely hear about it.

The human body cannot excrete alcohol; it has to be converted into acetaldehyde by the liver, and then the acetaldehyde can be excreted. This is the nasty substance that can give us a headache the day after a big night. If the liver didn't do its job properly and alcohol has accumulated in our blood, we can go into a coma and die. Alcohol is that poisonous. And I don't say that lightly. But, thankfully, our liver jumps into action and starts the conversion process and we carry on. Over time, though, this can take its toll. The trouble is, when we drink daily, or for some just regularly, the liver can be so busy dealing with alcohol as its priority that other substances that the liver has to change so they can be excreted don't get any attention and are recycled. Estrogen and cholesterol are two examples. It is often the reabsorption of these substances that leads to their elevated levels in our bodies — and that can lead to health challenges.

FOR WOMEN...
NO MORE THAN
two
STANDARD DRINKS
PER DAY WITH
two
ALCOHOL-FREE DAYS
PER WEEK

Many people start thinking about their first drink earlier in the day, and often when they arrive home they are thirsty and hungry. If you want to cut back or cut out alcohol for a while, or even if you just want to break your habit of regular drinking, have a big glass of water when you first get home and notice whether that takes the edge off your desire for alcohol. Most alcoholic drinks contain high levels of sugars, and so have a snack that contains some wholefood fats and see if that alleviates your desire for alcohol.

For others, it is the ritual they link to their drinks. When you arrive home, still pour yourself a drink at the time you would normally have a glass of wine and do what you would normally do. Sit and chat to your partner, make dinner, talk on the phone to a friend. So often we have mentally linked the glass of wine to a pleasurable activity when it is actually the pleasurable activity that we don't want to miss out on! So have sparkling water in a wine glass, with some fresh lime or lemon if that appeals, and add a few more alcohol-free days to your life.

On the plus side, the Blue Zone work that studies the populations of the world who live to ripe old ages still highly functional (as opposed to reliant on others for services due to health problems) have found that one of the factors these groups have in common is that they tend to have a glass of wine at about 5pm, with friends. Did they squash the grapes to make the wine with their own feet? Possibly. Did they add preservative (a liver-loader) to the wine? No. Did they get drunk? No. Are they engaged in conversations that matter to them with people who matter to them while they drink? Yes.

If you drink alcohol, take a leaf out of the way of life of the Blue Zones populations.

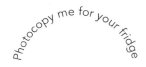

CHECK YOURSELF:

• KEEP IT UP •

Next time you pour a glass of wine, measure how much you pour and compare it to the guidelines in this article	
When you get home in the evening, instead of reaching for a glass of alcohol, start with a big drink of water and a satiating snack such as a handful of macadamia nuts and see if your desire for alcohol decreases	
Add a few more alcohol free days to your life – don't let alcohol dull your greatness	
Take some time to journal about what alcohol truly means to you and get honest with yourself about how it affects you – both while you're consuming and in the days that follow	

A STANDARD DRINK:

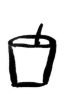 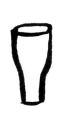  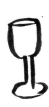

SPIRITS	BEER (4%)	CHAMPAGNE	WINE
30 mLs	**330 mLs**	**170 mLs**	**100 mLs**

BO

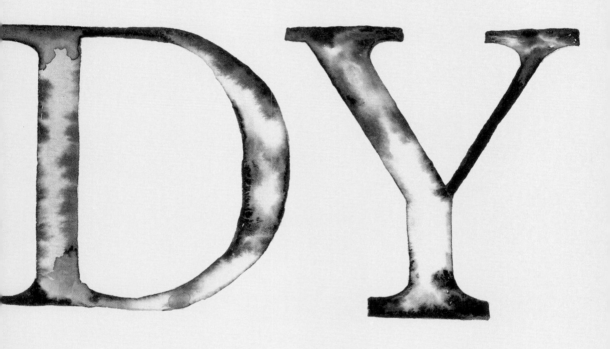

Your body is a gift to you. You can't trade it in, the way you might a car. This is it. And it doesn't have a voice, but it will give you symptoms to let you know whether it is happy or not. It is up to us to decipher them. And then act on them.

What if the parts of your body that sadden or frustrate you are simply messengers, asking you to eat, drink, move, sleep, think, breathe, believe or perceive in a new way?

See them as the gifts that they are.

skin

WHY WHAT WE PUT ON OUR SKIN MATTERS

Your skin is not simply a layer, it is an organ, and it is also a wonderful barometer of what is going on inside your body. All skin conditions, from rashes to acne to signs of aging, are the manifestations of your body's internal needs, including its nutritional ones.

The skin performs a multitude of tasks, most of which go unnoticed and under-appreciated. It protects us from disease and our daily exposure to particles in the air. It cools us when we are hot, and warms us when we are cold. It heals wounds inflicted on it, often without any assistance from us. It absorbs sunlight and produces vitamin D, which is critical to our bones and teeth, it keeps itself moist, slows its own aging, and every day attempts to renew and restore itself. While skin accomplishes all of this on its own, it still needs support in order to thrive, not just function. As Susan West Kurz so beautifully describes in her book, *Awakening Beauty*, with every blemish, rash and wrinkle, the skin is asking us to understand its nature, and support its efforts at self-renewal. Unfortunately, many of us respond to changes in our skin with practices that actually assault and injure it further, consequently accelerating the aging process, whether that is visible immediately or not. Still others do nothing for their skin, but nonetheless expect it to remain clear, beautiful and youthful.

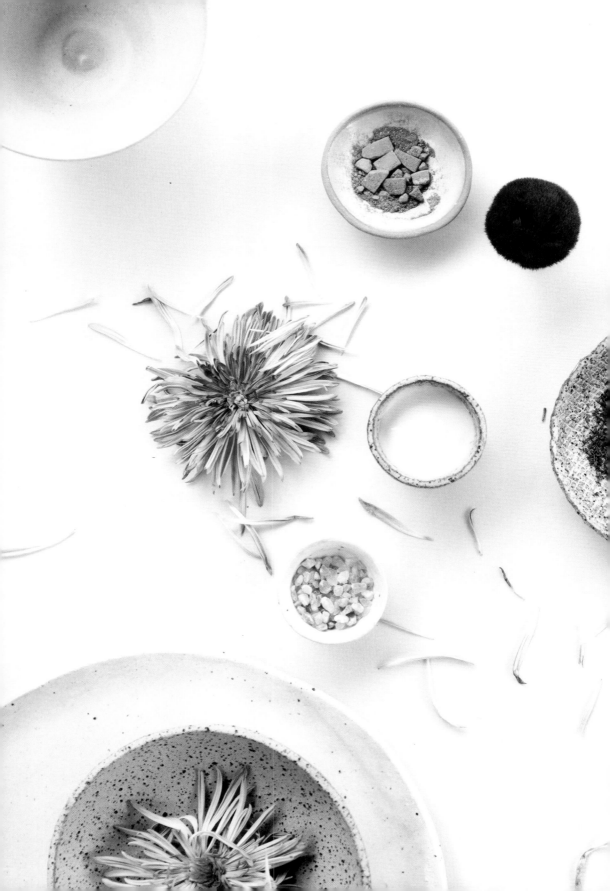

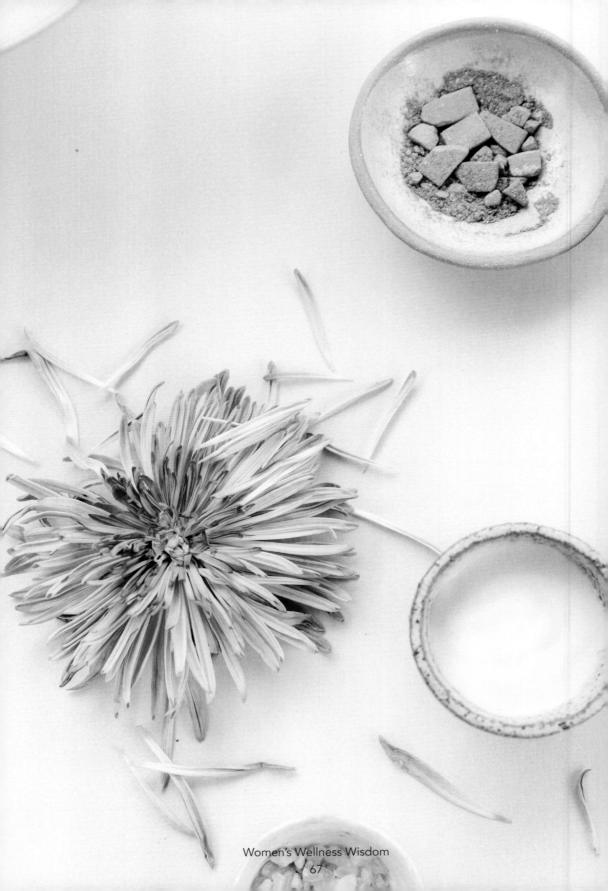

To help people change the way they consider and therefore treat their skin, I find it most powerful to help people understand what the skin does each day, and how best to support its work. Skin is actually made up of three layers, which together are the perfect shield. The outermost layer, which is renewed each month, is the epidermis and this is the part you can see. The middle layer is the dermis, which plays a critical role in how hydrated the skin is (I call the dermis "water world"), and below that is the foundation layer of the skin, known as the subcutaneous layer. All three layers work together to form healthy, vibrant skin.

The skincare you choose needs to help support the function and action of the skin (the organ), not suffocate or interfere with it. Plus, you want any products to be made from ingredients that don't add to the load of the detoxification mechanisms in your body. You can help decrease the synthetic chemical load in your life by considering what you put on your skin. You only have to think about how nicotine patches work to realize that your skin is a direct route to your blood supply, and that your detoxification systems will have additional work to do depending on what ends up in there. There are some beautiful skincare companies who create highly effective products that contain zero synthetic ingredients. Ideally, you want the ingredients to be certified organic or biodynamically grown. That way your skincare looks after you, and your choices help look after the planet.

Outer reflections

WHAT IS YOUR BODY TRYING TO TELL YOU?

What are some of the common "surface" symptoms trying to attract your attention? Here is my take on what I have seen work with some common "beauty" challenges. When you want to alter something on the outside, it helps to remember that it is usually the inside that created it. Eczema is a great example. It appears on the skin yet it is almost always resolved with dietary change.

EYES AND AROUND THE EYES

Dark circles

Focus on digestion and/or liver support. Based on what you have learnt in this book and what has welled up for you, trial either a dairy-free diet or a gluten-free diet for four weeks to see whether it makes a difference. I have seen both dietary trials resolve dark circles. Liver herbs can also be beneficial.

Dry eyes or floaters in vision

Focus on liver support. Check for iron deficiency as well.

Puffy eyes

Adrenal support is very important. Drink only water or herbal tea for two weeks (ie, no other drinks) and see whether this makes a difference.

Thinning outer-third of eyebrow

Focus particularly on thyroid support. It would be wise to have some thyroid tests done. However, remember that if they show up in the "normal" range they may be skewed one way, and in this case you need to treat the signs that your body is giving you, rather than the blood results. Work with an experienced practitioner to do this.

HAIR AND SCALP

Brittle hair

Support your thyroid and adrenals, and increase your intake of essential fatty acids (EFAs) and vitamin C.

Dandruff / flaky scalp

This can be a vitamin A deficiency, an EFA deficiency, or gut dysbiosis. If you believe that for you it is more likely to be the last option, and that there are some less-than-friendly bacterial species living in your large intestine, trial a diet where you eat zero refined sugar, and eat carbs only from wholefood sources, such as root vegetables. Trial this initially for four weeks, and, if you feel there is an improvement, continue for a total of three months to assess whether it will resolve within this period. You might also like to add more coconut to your diet, as the lauric acid in it may also assist the scalp. Rubbing coconut oil into your scalp the evening before you wash your hair can also help. Amp up the greens and the wholefood fat in your diet as well.

Hair loss

Support your thyroid and adrenals, and look at your sex hormone balance and vitamin D status.

Hairy chin, facial hair

This is often due to increased levels of androgens in the skin. Start with stress hormone management strategies, including breath-focused restorative practices. When darkened facial hair has started to appear, it is very important for these girls or women to learn how to live from a calm place, not just accessing a calm place when they do yoga and then go back to living with adrenal-depleting intensity.

LIPS AND AROUND THE MOUTH

Bad breath

Focus on resolving any gut or digestion challenges.

Chapped lips

Focus on digestive system support, and support stomach acid production, using lemon juice in warm water or apple cider vinegar.

Cracks at the corners of the mouth

This can be due to a B vitamin deficiency (usually riboflavin, vitamin B2), an iron deficiency, or both.

Teeth strength and prevention of cavities

Minerals such as calcium, magnesium, manganese, boron and vitamin D all strengthen teeth. If you notice significant changes to your teeth, consider seeing a holistic dentist, focus on a refined-sugar-free, mineral-rich way of eating, and explore the need for adrenal support. Brush twice daily. Floss. Smile.

NAILS

Dull nails

This can indicate poor diet, poor digestion, or a folate deficiency, especially if you are on the oral contraceptive pill. Amp up your greens, along with supporting digestion, via chewing well, stimulating stomach acid production (apple cider vinegar) and drinking water between meals, rather than with meals.

Lined nails — grooves across the nail

Adrenal support may be needed, and restorative practices are essential.

Lined nails — grooves from base to tip

This can indicate a mineral deficiency, such as calcium and/or magnesium. It can also indicate that the thyroid needs support.

Pale, brittle, withered or weak nails

Liver support is necessary; it can also indicate an iron deficiency. If your dietary iron intake is good, have iron blood studies done to determine whether a deficiency exists. If so, explore why. "Unexplained" iron deficiency can highlight digestive system challenges or coeliac disease.

Peeling or scabby cuticles

This can be due to iron deficiency, EFA deficiency, or sympathetic nervous system (SNS) dominance. Apply the appropriate strategy or strategies. Also try a rubbing a little coconut oil around your nail beds each evening.

Soft nails

Make sure you are getting adequate dietary protein. If you are sure that you are, focus on digestive system support. To make keratin, a tough protein that is a major component in hard, strong nails, the body needs high-quality protein and good stomach acid production.

Spoon-shaped nails

This is often due to iron deficiency. There may also be deficiencies in vitamin B12 and/or folate.

White spots on nails

This typically indicates a zinc deficiency.

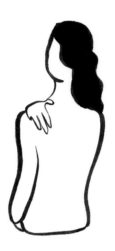

SKIN

Back-ne

Quite often a sex hormone imbalance perpetuates this, arising from high levels of androgens in the skin, elevated prolactin, or an imbalance between estrogen and progesterone. All of these situations can be tested for if the condition is ongoing or if it doesn't respond to the sex hormone balancing suggestions, including liver support. The first place I start with is stress management, due to the role cortisol plays in the conversion of other hormones to androgens, alongside liver support.

Body odour

This is usually a call for additional liver support.

Bumps on the backs of arms

This can be the result of an EFA deficiency and/or due to excess fruit consumption. If EFAs are supplemented, including evening primrose oil in the mix can be helpful. If that doesn't work, explore whether you might be zinc-deficient.

Cellulite

Liver and lymphatic support has been shown to decrease the appearance of cellulite. Rebounding is a wonderful way to stimulate the lymphatic system. Significantly limiting or omitting liver-loaders has also been shown to reduce the appearance of cellulite, or in some cases even allows it to disappear. Good-quality herbal medicine can also be highly beneficial, particularly St Mary's thistle and globe artichoke.

Cold sores

Cold sores are caused by the herpes virus, so immune support is vital: consider consuming additional vitamin C and zinc, and some immune support herbs. Herpes only reactivates itself when you trigger it with stress, poor dietary choices, or too little sleep. Herpes is like a seed in a desert: it will stay asleep indefinitely if the signal to germinate isn't given. It is also important to minimize intake of foods that can feed viruses, such as reducing dietary exposure to the amino acid arginine. When the amino acid lysine is higher in your diet than the amino acid arginine, herpes has trouble replicating. When arginine is higher than lysine, herpes multiplies quickly. Foods high in arginine include chocolate, crustaceans, soy and peanuts.

Cracked elbows

This indicates an EFA deficiency and/or zinc deficiency.

Cracked heels

This often indicates a deficiency in EFAs.

Dry skin

This may indicate an EFA deficiency, poor skincare choice, thyroid dysfunction, poor diet or poor digestion.

Eczema in adults

Follow a strict dairy-free diet trial for four weeks. If that doesn't make a difference at all, bring dairy back, and omit all red foods, such as chillies, capsicums (peppers), tomatoes, strawberries, apples (red and green), for a four-week trial and see whether that makes a difference. Or, if you eat more than two pieces of fruit a day, cut back to less than two, or omit fruit for a trial period of four weeks to see whether that makes a difference. An evening primrose oil supplement can also be highly beneficial, as it contains an enzyme called delta-6-desaturase, which allows fat to be incorporated into the skin, keeping it moist and youthful. For chronic, widespread adult eczema, I encourage you to also explore the metaphysical basis of adult eczema — rage toward a masculine figure in your life.

Fluid accumulation at the ankles

This indicates that the liver and/or the kidneys need support. Do a four-week trial omitting caffeine; most people will notice a significant decrease in the fluid accumulation at the ankles in particular. You may also need herbal liver support.

Newly oily skin and/or oily scalp

If greasy skin or a greasy scalp is new for you, it may signal that your sex hormones are imbalanced. This is particularly likely to be the case if you notice the greasiness increases in the lead-up to menstruation. Utilize the sex hormone support strategies discussed throughout the book to see if that makes a difference.

Oily skin at the same time as dry skin

Work on supporting sex hormone production; in particular, make sure that the pituitary gland is talking to the ovaries and that ovulation is occurring. Vitex can offer lovely support, as can paeonia and licorice taken together. Combination skin can also be a sign that the liver needs some love. Skincare may need to be changed to better support the skin's functioning.

Pale, grey-tinged, dull skin

This can be a sign of poor nutrition from poor food choices, or of poor digestion. Focus on eating more real-food if you don't already, and/or support your digestion through stress management, eating slowly, chewing food well, and drinking water between meals, rather than with meals.

Pigmentation on the face newly appearing

This can indicate a sex hormone imbalance; typically too much estrogen. Apply sex hormones balancing information based on other symptoms related to your cycle.

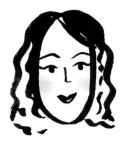

Pimples and blemishes on the jawline

This can be a sign that your sex hormones need support. Do a dairy-free trial for four weeks, plus support good gut and liver health.

Psoriasis

Avoid pork and tomatoes for a trial period of four weeks. EFA supplementation can be beneficial, as can additional zinc. Enquire within to see whether there was a time in your life when you decided to "thicken your skin" to avoid emotional hurts.

Redness on the face; flushing easily

Commit to a dairy-free diet trail for four weeks.

Rosacea

Support the liver, and follow a strict dairy-free diet trial for a minimum of four weeks. You will notice significantly less redness by the end of this trial period if you are going to respond. EFAs can also be highly beneficial.

Scars

Consider taking additional vitamin C and/or zinc. Using lavender oil and/or calendula oil can also be beneficial to decreasing the appearance of scars.

Stretch marks

They often indicate a zinc deficiency, past or present. You can also use lavender oil to help minimize their appearance.

Skin challenges

WHY DO YOU HAVE CHALLENGES EVEN THOUGH YOU'RE AN ADULT?

Have you ever wondered, if you experience challenges with your skin, why this might be so? Here are some questions I have been asked over the years, the answers to which I hope offer you some insights you can apply to your life, if required.

What types of foods in our diet cause blemishes, specifically on our chin?

The face is a useful tool for exploring deeper issues. Flare-ups of pimples, acne, rosacea, eczema and rashes are a signal that other body systems may not be functioning at their best. More often than not it is the gut that is not as happy as it could be. Poor digestion can lead to overloaded liver detoxification pathways that then struggle to clear unwanted substances from the body. When these substances are not eliminated efficiently, the body looks for another way to excrete them, and the skin is then used as an excretory organ. This can trigger pimples and other skin troubles. A diet high in plant foods and plenty of water, and avoiding caffeine, trans fats, processed sugars and alcohol, can all contribute to good digestion and happy, radiant, clear skin.

Almost always, poor digestive function is the first trigger for acne. Poor digestion adds a load to the liver and kidneys; they aren't able to filter the higher levels of hormones in the blood efficiently, and the hormones stimulate additional sebum production. I have seen countless cases of acne improve and then resolve with a commitment to caring for and supporting the digestive system, liver and kidneys; essentially, the waste-disposal units of the body.

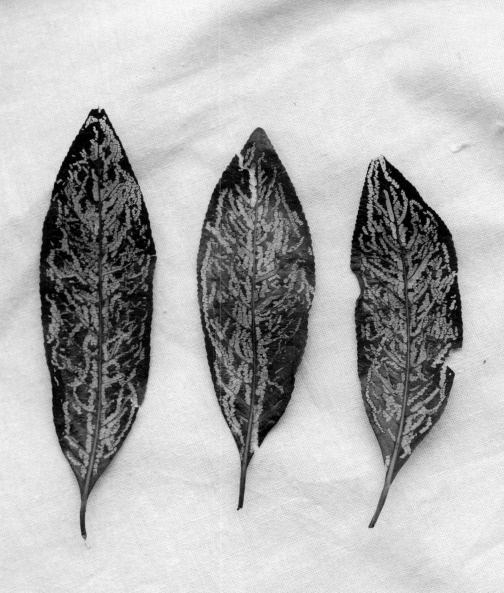

What should we eat more of, and less of, to avoid those big nasty cystic acne bumps on our chin?

Although scientific evidence pertaining to the effectiveness of a nourishing diet on many skin conditions is limited, in my clinical experience many skin conditions, including cystic acne, respond well to a reduction or elimination of refined sugars in the diet, likely due to the impact less sugar has on changing gut bacteria profiles. Clinically, the other dietary change I have seen make a difference to cyst formation on the chin for some people is a dairy-free diet. This must be super-strict for the trial period, and you need to read food labels to ensure this occurs. A health professional can guide you with this.

Many people also respond well to a diet rich in essential fatty acids, good fats such as avocado, nuts and seeds, and plenty of leafy green vegetables. Foods rich in vitamin C and zinc are also beneficial, due to their healing and immune system properties. The richest food source of zinc is oysters. Beef and lamb also contain some, and our plant sources include seeds, such as sunflower seeds and pumpkin seeds. Foods high in vitamin C include berries, capsicums (peppers), citrus fruits, kale and parsley.

For clear, beautiful skin, do we need to avoid inflammatory foods? Such as...

Start by eating real-food. Real-food, as it comes in nature, is packed with a range of nutrients, all of which promote great skin. Avoid processed food, caffeine and alcohol, and then notice the difference this makes to your skin. Vitamin C is particularly helpful for skin, as it helps to combat free radical damage, which is part of the cause of aging and wrinkles. Vitamin C also helps build collagen and helps to prevent its breakdown, supporting the skin's elasticity and youthful appearance. Vitamin C-rich foods include citrus fruit, kiwifruit, capsicum and broccoli.

Skin loves fat! Fat helps the skin to maintain its moisture barrier, which helps keep skin soft and prevents drying. Flaky and dry skin or cracked heels and cuticles can be a sign that you are lacking in essential fatty acids.

The anti-inflammatory omega-3 fatty acids are particularly helpful for skin, and are the type of fat that most people are deficient in. Oily fish, like sustainable sardines or salmon, and chia seeds, flax seeds and walnuts are all great omega-3-rich fats to include in your diet. Minimizing the inflammation-driving omega-6 fats found in many processed foods is also important. Coconut oil also makes a great topical moisturizer to use on dry patches of skin.

How do we know what foods might be causing our skin to breakout? Do we need to do an elimination diet?

An elimination diet can be very helpful if you are noticing triggers around the consumption of particular foods. This is particularly relevant for skin conditions such as eczema or psoriasis. However, elimination diets are best done under the guidance of a qualified health professional to ensure you don't miss out on vital nutrition. I would recommend keeping a food diary as the first action step, to take note of any flare-ups pertaining to the consumption of particular foods. It is also important to note

if skin flare-ups are related to your menstrual cycle, as this can indicate that liver detoxification pathways need additional support.

In a nutshell, healthy adult skin needs:

- real-food
- food gut health
- efficient liver detoxification — herbal medicine can be a wonderful support for this
- good hydration — make water your main drink
- essential fats
- vitamin C and zinc
- balanced sex hormones: as you will learn elsewhere in this book, the three most common scenarios of sex hormone imbalance are excess estrogen, low progesterone and no progesterone:
  - excess estrogen: liver support is required
  - low progesterone: ovarian follicle nutrients can help, such as iodine, selenium, vitamin D and zinc
  - no progesterone: the goal is to get you ovulating regularly, and useful herbs include paeonia, licorice and vitex.

Beautiful filtration

SUPPORT YOUR KIDNEYS, SUPPORT YOUR SKIN

One of the primary jobs of the kidneys is to remove the waste products of protein metabolism from the blood. These include nitrogen, uric acid (urea) and ammonia. The kidneys also remove many other substances from the blood that could become problematic if left to accumulate, including excess hormones, food additives, vitamins, minerals and drugs. They also regulate the electrolyte balance of the body, which involves the minerals needed for healthy nerve function. These include calcium, magnesium, phosphate, sodium, potassium and chloride. The kidneys also help regulate healthy blood pressure.

The kidneys regulate the amount of water in the body, and your urine is what remains after your blood has been filtered by the kidneys. Water plays an enormous role in keeping the moisture content of our skin at a lovely high level. Consuming adequate water also helps to promote healthy waste elimination, and it reduces the likelihood of constipation, as one of the primary functions of the large intestine is to absorb water from digested food. When water consumption is low, stools tend to become dry, hard and more difficult to pass, and the longer this waste remains inside the body, the more waste will be reabsorbed back into the bloodstream, through which it soon finds its way to the skin.

It is obvious, then, that if we are to have beautiful, well-hydrated skin, as well as great overall health, we must take good care of our kidneys.

On the following page are some tips on how to support their optimal function.

Drink adequate amounts of pure water each day.

Keep a large glass at your desk to ensure you stay hydrated over the day. Let your body guide you on how much water it needs by noticing your response to the water you drink. As you drink, observe whether your thirst becomes awakened and your body actually seems to draw in the water. This is your body letting you know that it needs more water. Sometimes you might start drinking and want another glass immediately. At other times, you are satisfied with one glass or just a few sips. Give your body all the water it needs throughout the day to ensure that the elimination of waste via the urine is well-supported. It is also important to omit (or certainly minimize) your consumption of soft drinks, and be honest with yourself about how much alcohol you are consuming. Every day is too much. If you have any type of skin condition, this is even more critical, and is particularly important for children and teenagers.

Sleep well!

You will notice that when you are exhausted, not only does everything feel more difficult, but your skin is also less radiant and more prone to breakouts, blemishes and rashes. Rest and sleep strengthen the kidneys. Seven to nine hours of restorative sleep per night allows the kidneys to adequately cleanse the blood, eliminating waste products in the morning urine that would otherwise be shunted to the skin for excretion. Do all you can to establish a consistent rhythm between your sleeping and waking hours, particularly if you would like more vitality. Consider taking a short nap on the weekends, especially when you are going through times of stress, which for many people these days is every week!

Take part in regular restorative movement such as t'ai chi, qi gong, yoga and/or restorative yoga.

These practices not only have specific poses or movements to support healthy kidney function, but the diaphragmatic breathing they foster is a powerful tool to decrease stress hormone production, which is essential for optimal health.

Hair

WHY IS YOUR HAIR FALLING OUT?

Have you noticed that you experience times of what seems like major hair loss, and then others it seems to be more moderate or even non-existent? A certain amount of hair loss is supposed to happen, and new hair grows. However, what is becoming more and more common is how many women now experience significant hair loss at some stage in their lives. At times, this is temporary and it occurs for only a few months, often following a period of major change or stress. Yet for others, major hair loss is continuous.

How do you know if you are losing too much hair? When a significant amount of hair has been lost, you will notice your part becoming wider and there will be hair on your pillow most, if not every, morning.

If this is something you are experiencing, the most common causes of significant female hair loss include:

- iron deficiency
- poor thyroid function or thyroid disease
- polycystic ovarian syndrome (PCOS)
- hormonal contraception or replacement therapy
- pregnancy
- after childbirth
- autoimmune alopaecia, and
- chronic illness.

However, if all of the above are tested for, yet no cause is found for your hair loss, it can leave you wondering what to do to resolve it. You may start to believe that it must be genetic because you haven't found any other explanation. Sure, genetic predisposition can play a role in all health conditions, but epigenetics has taught us that it is the environment (of which diet is a part) that pulls the trigger. In other words, it is lifestyle choices that drive the genes to express themselves or not.

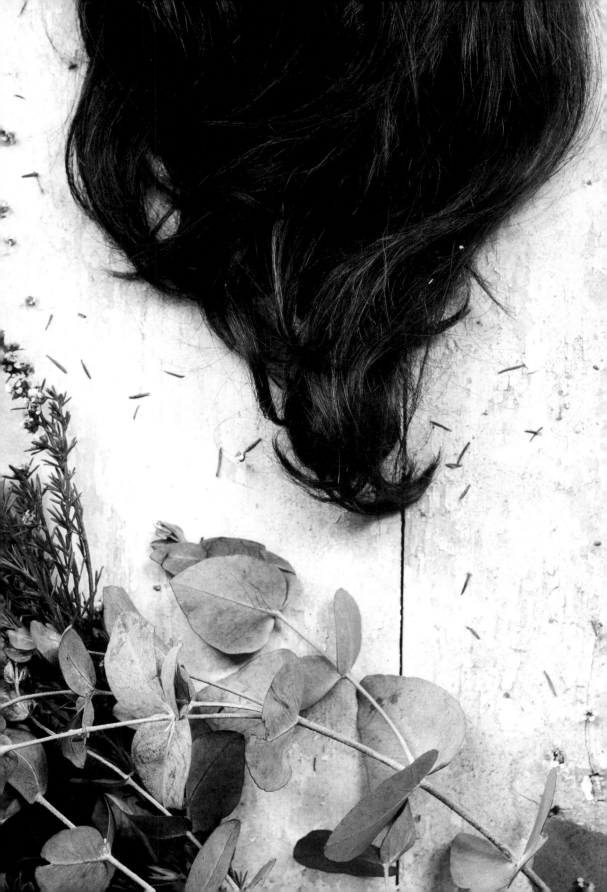

So what are some of the factors in the modern world that might be contributing to hair loss? Over two decades of working with women, I have found that hair loss in women is commonly not due to disease but to sex hormones. Sometimes this has involved some type of hormonal-based contraception — pills, implants or injections. Other times, cycle changes indicated that innate sex hormones ratios had changed.

When a hormonally-based contraception method was in use, what these methods tended to have in common was a synthetic form of progesterone known as "progestin", which can behave like testosterone in the body. Progestins are referred to as "androgenic" (testosterone is an androgen), and they have been shown to shrink hair follicles. Hair loss stemming from these synthetic hormones can take a long time — years even — to become noticeable.

Another feature of significant female hair loss that I have observed in practice over the years is the elevation of markers (in the blood) of chronic inflammation, often generated by lifestyle factors such as a poor-quality diet, smoking and/or chronic stress. Dietary change, nutritional supplementation and herbal medicine are typically highly effective at lowering these inflammatory markers, with hair improvements evident after about three to six months.

When the basis of the hair loss was naturally elevated androgens (not from contraception), both liver and adrenal support were needed, along with stress management techniques, such as restorative practices.

If significant hair loss is something that is occurring for you, please first see your GP and have the medical conditions listed above investigated.

Here are some general tips to help support healthy hair when much has been lost. Keep in mind that your hair can take some time to improve, as your hair today tends to be a reflection of your health three to six months ago. So be patient.

Support healthy hair

- Work to balance sex hormone levels so that estrogen is high when it is supposed to be, and progesterone is high when it is supposed to be, ensuring regular ovulation and a regular menstrual cycle. If this is not currently occurring, refer to the pieces about estrogen and progesterone, elsewhere in this book, as liver, adrenal, ovarian and/or pituitary support is often needed.

- Ensure you are eating in a way that is right for you. Use the information from the "Eat" section to help guide you with this. Do you digest dairy or gluten well? Avoid food sensitivities, because if you aren't digesting a food well, it can contribute to inflammation.

- Eat real-food. Avoid deep-fried foods and refined sugars and starches, preservatives and artificial colours, and sweeteners. Just eat real-food. Ensure that what you eat is rich in plants, as plant foods contain substances unique to each plant that help liver detoxification, immune function, and substances that help to decrease inflammation. The Just Eat Real-Food approach overall helps to decrease inflammation, as well as giving you the nutrients you need for great hair health.

- Have your zinc and iron levels ("iron studies") tested by your GP. If they are low, they must be replenished with diet and/or nutritional supplements. Zinc and iron are both needed for healthy hair follicles, and they are the two most common nutritional deficiencies in the Western world, particularly among women of menstruation age. Food sources of zinc include oysters (very high level), red meat (moderate amount) and seeds (low level). Food sources of iron include red meat (highly bioavailable iron), eggs (moderate), green vegies and dates (lower levels).

- Promote good digestion, particularly the gut bacteria. They can create or lower inflammation, and every other body system relies on the optimal functioning of the gut.

- Consult your GP or medical specialist about potentially choosing a different type of birth control method that does not contain an androgenic progestin, or explore the use of non-hormonal methods of contraception.

Thyroid troubles

COULD THIS BE YOU?

Thyroid dysfunction and thyroid diseases are on the rise across the Western world. You don't have to have a thyroid disease for poor thyroid function to affect your health in a lousy way. Here's how we start to work it out.

DIAGNOSIS

First, please note that many of the symptoms of an overactive thyroid are often the opposite of an underactive thyroid, but some people may experience both conditions in their lifetime.

Symptoms of an overactive thyroid include:

- "unexplained" weight loss
- over-heating easily
- tendency to "unexplained" loose stools
- rapid heartbeat or heart palpitations
- amped-up regularly with a tendency to feel anxious
- eyes bulging forward from the eye sockets
- chronic stress
- family history of thyroid dysfunction or disease
- family history of autoimmune conditions
- diagnosis of adrenal fatigue or another condition involving the endocrine system, or previous diagnosis of an autoimmune condition.

Symptoms of an underactive thyroid include:

- "unexplained" weight gain

- feeling cold in your bones, or you notice you are colder than others around you — you are the first to put on a jumper

- when you read about the symptoms of an underactive thyroid, they resonate with you, even though you have been told that your blood test results are fine; when you see them, though, the results tend to be skewed to one end of the "normal" range

- a tendency to constipation, dry skin, brittle hair

- long-term estrogen-dominance symptoms, such as premenstrual syndrome

- bone-weariness; you are beyond tired

- body feels heavy and lethargic

- reactions to stimuli (both physical and emotional) feel slow

- craving for salt

- craving coffee, but it doesn't amp you up, although your brain feels slightly more functional after you have it

- groin aches

- change in voice: it is husky on occasions, particularly when you are extra tired (this can also be a sign that the adrenals need support)

- feeling like you are retaining fluid

- tendency to a depressed mood, forgetfulness and a sense of being easily confused

- hair loss

- difficulty conceiving

- challenges with menstruation

- recurrent headaches

- gallbladder has been removed

- chronic stress

- family history of thyroid dysfunction or disease

- family history of autoimmune conditions

- diagnosis of adrenal fatigue or another condition involving the endocrine system, or previous diagnosis of an autoimmune condition

- sense of wondering when it will be your turn; when will you be able to do what you want to do, rather than what others want or need from you.

Based on your symptoms, if you also have:

- elevated thyroid-stimulating hormone (TSH) or high-end of normal TSH
- low or low-end of normal thyroxine (T4) levels

then you may need thyroid support for an underactive thyroid.

If you also have auto-antibodies to your thyroid gland, then you may be diagnosed with Hashimoto's thyroiditis.

Or, based on your symptoms, if you also have:

- low or low-end of normal TSH
- high or high-end of normal T4

then you may need support for an overactive thyroid.

If you also have auto-antibodies to your thyroid gland, then you may be diagnosed with Graves' disease.

Underlying causes, and treatment. Things that interfere with good thyroid function include:

- iodine deficiency
- iron deficiency
- selenium deficiency
- insulin resistance, leading to the body becoming "deaf" to leptin
- estrogen dominance
- poor liver detoxification processes
- chronic stress.

To work out the method of treatment and support for you, we need to know what caused the thyroid dysfunction in the first place. The road in shows us the road we need to take out. For example, if your thyroid isn't working properly because of iodine deficiency, then repleting your iodine levels will restore thyroid function. However, if your thyroid isn't working properly because of long-term estrogen dominance, then no amount of iodine will correct that — resolving the estrogen dominance will improve thyroid function.

Solutions that may be suitable, depending on what has created poor thyroid function in you, include:

- going on a grain-free diet trial for a minimum of four weeks — gut health often needs to be at the heart of thyroid treatments, particularly if there are antibodies present in the blood

- going on a four-week dairy-free trial if you love dairy products and the idea of going without cheese makes you wonder if you could; it is often what we love (not just like) to eat that can be a problem

- having an experienced health professional assess your diet for iodine and selenium intake, and having a blood test to examine not only thyroid parameters, but also iron status

- supporting liver and gallbladder function to assist with bowel elimination (globe artichoke is particularly good for "thyroid" people)

- referring to the advice about estrogen dominance, elsewhere in this book

- supporting the adrenals — this is almost always essential, especially when beginning to treat the thyroid (ideas are scattered through this book, and include regular, restorative practices)

- taking a four-week break from coffee, if you crave coffee, and observe how you feel at the end of this period — drink green tea, which has a lower caffeine level, herbal tea, or dandelion tea instead

- exploring transitioning to whole thyroid extract under medical supervision, if you have a diagnosed thyroid condition and you are on synthetic medication but your symptoms are still present.

Stress express

THE NERVOUS SYSTEM – A BODY SYSTEM TO REALLY UNDERSTAND

We are wired for survival. We will do more to avoid pain than we will ever do to have pleasure. It has to be this way for all animals. Otherwise, a species would die out. And it is via the nervous system that so much information is conveyed throughout the body: if signals are sent that indicate that your life is in danger, the body has no choice but to respond accordingly.

This means that in modern times many people spend all day, most days, on red alert, and this can impact on many body systems and parts, including:

- the fuel your body believes is "safe" and appropriate to use in that moment
- how your clothes fit you
- the quality of your sleep
- your digestion, and whether your tummy is comfortable or is regularly bloated
- your blood pressure
- your eyesight
- blood glucose regulation
- hunger signals
- satiety signals
- food cravings
- regular energy crashes
- mood fluctuations.

Here's what you need to know about the nervous system, and to help you get clear about some lifestyle choices you might like to make. This will help you signal to your body that it is "safe", and therefore allow efficient body fat utilization, among these other things, particularly related to the relationship between stress and body fat.

THE AUTONOMIC NERVOUS SYSTEM

Everything in our internal and external environments — including the food we eat, the exercise we do (or don't do) and the thoughts we think — influences our nervous system. When it comes to weight management, people believe that in order to become healthy they must lose some weight. I believe the opposite is true: in order to lose weight, we must become healthy, and I approach weight loss for clients in this way.

To understand this, we need to explore how the autonomic nervous system (ANS) works. The autonomic nervous system "runs" our body behind the scenes and is not under our conscious control. It regulates our heart rate, respiration rate, temperature control, and immune and hormonal systems while we carry on with life. Don't you think it is truly miraculous that if you cut yourself the wound just heals? Don't you think it is amazing that you swallow food and your digestive system extracts the nutrients to nourish you so you can stay alive? To say that the human body is extraordinary is an understatement!

There are three parts to the autonomic nervous system. They are the sympathetic nervous system (SNS), the parasympathetic nervous system (PNS) and the enteric nervous system (ENS). Here, I will focus on the SNS, the "fight-or-flight" system, and the PNS, the "rest and repair" system, and their interaction.

In general, the SNS and the PNS have opposite functions. When the nervous system perceives that we are under "threat" — which in modern times can be due to caffeine consumption and/or our perception of pressure and urgency — the SNS raises our heart rate, increases our respiratory rate, releases stress hormones (adrenalin and cortisol) and shunts blood away from the digestive tract to the muscles so that we can run away from, or fight, whatever is threatening us. If organ systems in the body are unhealthy, and therefore stressed themselves, or if we are mentally or emotionally stressed, that increases the sympathetic load as well.

The SNS by its very nature is catabolic, meaning that it breaks down muscle tissue due to the increased amounts of secreted cortisol. High-intensity exercise is also sympathetic in nature; the heart rate goes up, as do respiration and body temperature, and cortisol is released into the blood. And, when in excess, cortisol increases body fat, amongst other things. Once the "threat" is dealt with (is it ever dealt with in the modern world?), the PNS slows our heart rate and respiration, and it brings the blood back to the digestive tract so that we can digest our food. It also works on repairing any tissues that have been damaged in our "battle", and allows libido to be restored (your survival instinct can't have you thinking about reproduction when your body believes that your life is being threatened).

Once the nervous system is better balanced, body fat is readily burned, a concept that is game-changing to the way you approach your body and your health.

The PNS is able to do its wonderful work overnight, provided we go to bed early enough, because cortisol naturally starts to rise around 2am. The SNS and the PNS are designed to balance each other. In people who have a well-balanced nervous system, high-intensity exercise tends to lead to fat loss because the parasympathetic rest time between workouts is when muscle tissue is built. The other metabolic and biochemical consequences of high-intensity exercise are, however, beyond the scope of this book.

It is likely that people who are unable to lose fat by doing regular high-intensity exercise have a dominant SNS, and, as a result, an inhibited PNS. In situations like this, because there is too much systemic stress coming from somewhere, adding high-intensity exercise is counterproductive. It adds to an individual's sympathetic load, exacerbating the nervous system imbalance. This is one of the reasons we have to get our heads around "it's not about the calories" when it comes to weight loss. If "burning" more of them has not solved your body fat challenge up until now, it is not suddenly going to start until some other work is done. And once the other work is done, you won't need to go back to sustained, high-intensity exercise and caloric deprivation to maintain your new level of health and energy, and the size and shape of your body.

Anxiety is so incredibly common today, often as a result of relationship challenges, financial stress, a poor diet and its consequences, worries about health or weight or whether you have upset someone, or simply the juggling act of life, worrying you might "let someone down". Yet, a person may be in sympathetic overload and still not even mention feeling anxious.

Reducing the sympathetic load is essential to great health and energy, as well as body fat loss, if the SNS is dominant. Movement is still important, but it is best approached from a different angle and with a different attitude. Far more effective exercise for SNS-dominant people are breath-focused restorative practices — exercise types such as t'ai chi, qi gong, yoga and Stillness Through Movement. These types of exercise significantly assist in increasing PNS activity via the breath, which helps balance the ANS. Building muscle is also critically important to (among other things) metabolic rate, and long-duration, high-intensity workouts tend to break muscle down, not build it. Once the nervous system is better balanced, body fat is readily burned — a concept that is game-changing to the way you approach your body and your health.

THE NERVOUS SYSTEM AND BODY FAT

In any given moment, the human body is making a decision about which fuel to use, based on the information it is receiving from the internal and external environments. The only two fuels for the human body are glucose (sugar) and fat — you don't use protein for fuel. The body breaks proteins down into amino acids, which are then converted into glucose so the body can use that glucose as fuel (energy). The name of this biochemical pathway is gluconeogenesis. The body requires energy for everything it does, from walking to sleeping, laughing to blinking; it all requires fuel.

As you now know, adrenalin communicates to every cell of your body that your life is in danger and prepares you to fight or flee. However, you may be making adrenalin simply because you have to make a phone call that you would rather not make, or perhaps because you have gulped down three cups of coffee already today. Or maybe your dad yelled at you a lot when you were a child, and so, even though you know now that your dad yelled a lot because that was how he communicated and coped with how stressed he felt (rather than it being about his lack of love for you), now when a male in your life raises his voice in your vicinity, you instinctively go into the "flight-or-fight" response. The majority of stress for most people in the Western world today is psychological rather than physical, and it can be constant and relentless.

The branch of the nervous system that is activated with stress of any type is the SNS, which has an intimate relationship with adrenalin. If the body's perception is that it needs to escape from impending danger, whether your thinking mind is telling you so or not, you need a fast-burning fuel available to allow you to do that. Your body thinks it has to get out of there and get out of there fast! So what fuel do you think your body will choose when it needs to flee, to get out of "danger" fast? Remember, its only choice is to burn either glucose or fat... In this scenario, it will choose predominantly glucose every time. The body thinks it has to in order to save our life, and we are all about survival. The body doesn't feel "safe" enough to use fat as its fuel in this "fight-or-flight" state, because fat offers us a steady, slow-release form of energy — not what we need in a time of danger. We can burn fat effectively in a PNS-dominant state, because the body perceives that it is safe when the PNS is activated. Yet, the PNS can never be the dominant arm of the ANS, it can never steer the ship while the body perceives there may be a threat to your life. This alone can be a significant block to a balanced nervous system, with the consequences impacting on all of the body systems listed at the beginning of this section, including utilizing body fat as a fuel and therefore leading to weight loss.

We have glucose stored in our muscles and liver in a form called "glycogen", and these stores are mobilized whenever our body gets the message that it needs energy to fight or run, if there is not enough glucose left in our blood from our last meal to fuel our escape. This mobilization of glycogen out of the muscles due to stress can, over time, impact on the function and appearance of our muscles, including allowing the onset of cellulite.

I believe that one of the most enormous health challenges of modern times is that the body can constantly be on the receiving end of the "fight-or-flight" messages. There are so many factors, internal and external to us, which drive this response within us that we have to begin to choose actively not to go there, not to get caught up in the rush. And to take steps in our daily lives to allow our nervous system to have some balance. Without this, using fat as a fuel — which gives us better and more consistent energy for a start — can be an uphill battle.

IN A NUTSHELL...

You want your body to move easily between SNS activation and PNS activation, not be "stuck" with the SNS activated all of the time.

To do this, you need to decrease SNS stimulation by:

- exploring how caffeine affects you — you may need to reduce your intake or take a break from it

- explore your perception of pressure and urgency and save it for when you really need it; for example, if you have to suddenly slam your brakes on while driving — not going through your email inbox.

You also want to actively activate the PNS. The only way science currently knows does this is by how you breathe, specifically by extending the length of your exhalation. That is partly why a breath-focused practice can be highly beneficial.

These include:

- yoga
- restorative yoga
- Stillness Through Movement
- pilates
- t'ai chi
- qi gong
- meditation

Or simply schedule time in your day, every hour on the hour, for example, to become breath-aware. Drop back down into belly-breathing if you find yourself chest-breathing.

Signs your nervous system needs support include:

- you feel stressed regularly, and feel that you are on red alert

- no matter how well you count calories and exercise, you struggle to lose weight (I'm not suggesting you count calories, but rather that you see this as a sign that stress may need to be addressed)

- you crave sugars and/or starches (carbohydrates)

- you love coffee, energy drinks — anything that contains caffeine — although sometimes you notice they make your heart race

- you startle (jump) easily

- you regularly don't sleep well

- you don't wake up feeling restored or with good energy

- if you don't go to sleep by 10pm, you get a second wind and end up staying awake until at least 1am

- you regularly feel tired but wired
- you are a worrier or a drama queen (or king)
- you feel anxious easily
- your breathing tends to be shallow and quite fast
- you experience "air hunger" (and other causes for this have been ruled out)
- you struggle to say "no"
- you laugh less than you used to
- you feel like everything is urgent
- you feel like there aren't enough hours in the day.

Ideas to help you better support your nervous system:

When you understand how your nervous system works, then you start to see what it needs, and I hope the following solutions will help you put that information to good use.

- embrace a restorative practice
- commit to a regular practice of diaphragmatic breathing
- instead of focusing on eating less sugar, focus on eating more dietary fats from wholefoods and/or green vegetables
- decrease or omit caffeine for four weeks (or two menstrual cycles if you experience PMT and/or period pain), and if you then feel much calmer, keep off the coffee, or switch from coffee to green tea, so that you consume smaller amounts of caffeine buffered by the effects of theanine in the green tea
- explore your perception of pressure and urgency. Have you made what you have to do each day full of pressure and urgency? Or is it a busy life, full of opportunity that is so ridiculously privileged because all of your basic needs are met? Of course there is real pressure and real urgency in this world, but save that perception for when you really need it, not for your everyday existence.

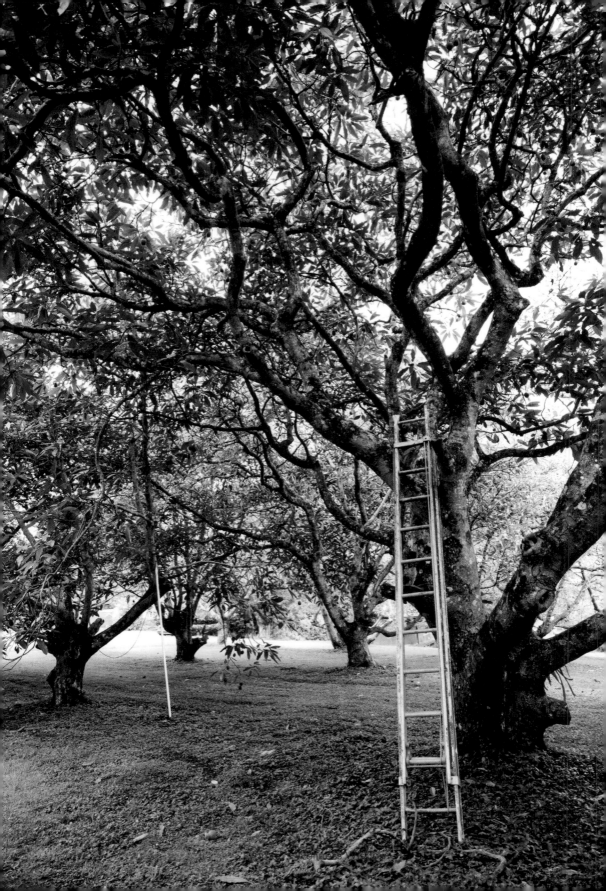

Shift your focus

FROM WEIGHT TO HEALTH AND ENERGY

I have witnessed countless people transform their bodies by relaxing and moving away from basing their food choices on the calorie equation. I have witnessed countless people go from eating a diet low in fat and high in complex carbohydrates, based on the food pyramid, and working hard doing five to seven cardiovascular gym workouts, in caloric deficit, and yet still constantly battling with their weight and experiencing weight fluctuations that they don't understand, and that the calorie equation cannot explain.

I have witnessed them shift to a whole real-food way of eating, much higher in fat, do resistance training, gentle forms of yoga, stretching, qi gong and/or walking; eating from 1200 to 2200 more calories per day than before, but not focusing on this, instead simply focusing on eating nourishing, nutrient-dense real whole foods. I have seen them lose weight, then stabilize their weight, and the results of any resistance work done in the gym are noticeable after one to two sessions, not months of hard slog. They never weigh themselves. Their clothes always fit. They have great energy and excellent health. Day after day. Year after year.

It is truly transformational when you shift your focus from weight and calories to health and nutrition. It is, after all, nutrients that keep us alive. And the better nourished we are, the better all of our inner processes (biochemical pathways) function, the better our digestion works, we sleep better, have better energy, and the happier we are.

Shift your focus to nourishing yourself.

"

If you get the inside right, the outside falls into place.

"

Digestive system & weight

IT'S NOT ABOUT THE CALORIES

Sometimes, when people first hear about my work, and they hear me say passionately that it is time to stop dieting, I get feedback that some people initially respond with something like "Oh, wow! She's saying not to diet. Yay! Eating rubbish or bingeing is fine — anything goes!" Yet I am not saying that, as they soon learn.

What deeply concerns me is that so many people feel that not dieting means bingeing, or living on poor-quality food. It tells me that people are used to depriving or shaming or punishing themselves as a way of life, and it is that approach to life I am really wanting to challenge. Since how you eat is how you live, deprivation as a way of treating yourself also shows up in how you eat.

For me, the real question I want to encourage you to explore is this: Do you feel the desire, the longing, to live in a different way? To live with ease and spaciousness. To stop punishing yourself or shaming yourself. Not only in your relationship with food, but in your relationship with other people, with work, with money and, most importantly, with yourself. And if you do, that gives you a choice about what to do, how to eat, what you focus your attention on, what your priorities are, how you perceive yourself, and how you live.

THREE-PRONGED HOLISTIC APPROACH TO HEALTH

To live in this different way requires a paradigm shift on how you approach what food you eat, and how you eat it. It requires a shift from a focus on weight to a genuine focus on and care for your health. This means embracing a three-pronged holistic approach to your health: emotion, nutrition and biochemistry. Let's explore these briefly here before we move on.

Emotion

1 When you are not hungry, it is not food you want. The food will never be enough, will never fill you, never satisfy you. Rather, it is the associations you have with the food, the stories you tell yourself about the food. It is the memories of that food. It is what you believe that eating that food will give you: a feeling — and it is always a feeling — of companionship, of belonging, of being welcomed, of no longer being lonely or bored, of being treasured, of deserving the sweet things in life, of being special. When you are not hungry, forget the middleman: food. Go for the treasuring. And start with yourself.

Nutrition

2 There is no question that humans can over-eat. Certainly it is very easy to do so in today's processed-food-laden world. It is also true that they can under-eat. However, the fundamental, underpinning problem is the way we are taught to approach eating: that the only way we can control or influence our body size and weight is via a concept of "calories in versus calories burned", which is based on an equation originating from 1918. This not only ignores the emotional factors that drive food behaviours (which are even more prevalent these days with the epidemic of "not enoughness" I talk about in my TEDx talk), but also ignores the dramatic change in our food supply. Since 1918, there has been a steady and remorseless

move away from real-food, contributing to what I call the "toxicity factor", and an influx of estrogen-like substances in the environment, which drives fat storage and disrupts our endocrine system.

3 Biochemistry

Couple this change in food source and content with the advent of the coffee culture, which can drive excess adrenalin production and promotes the fight-or-flight response. Then add to this our perceptions of pressure and urgency mounting daily, as evidenced by stress studies globally, and we have a whole host of factors influencing the metabolic consequences of the calories we eat. Fast-burning fuels are used over slower-burning fat, which is stored to help us survive these "unsafe" times. As this becomes our default setting, our metabolism changes.

The paradigm shift

When you base how someone is supposed to eat on a concept that says the only way you can have what you think you want — a slim body, a lean body — is by burning more than you eat, you set people up for a life of obsession and misery. Plus, you miss the road to freedom. By freeing yourself from an obsession with food and calories, from intense exercise, and from harsh self-talk, you will find what you seek from the food, but which it can never give you: love.

The body, mind and soul nourishing alternative is simple:

- eat real-food
- build your muscle mass
- get flexible
- diaphragmatically breathe
- drink mostly water
- get eight hours' sleep per night.

It is that simple. I always want to write "as often as you can" after these points, so that it feels more realistic for you. But the truth is, if I do that, you may not truly appreciate the powerful and wonderful impact a new level of commitment to your health and self-care can bring. I also always want to start points like these with a statement encouraging you to get back in touch with how precious life is, with how precious you are, for when you do that you will treat yourself accordingly. You will do these things without effort. Because that is part of what taking care of yourself looks like.

These points aren't rules. You do not need to follow them 24/7, 365 days a year. You are not required to execute them to perfection. It is what you consistently do that impacts on your health and your body. This is a way of life; a way of living you return to after a meal with a friend or a holiday. It is how we can support our body in this fast-paced modern world. It is how we can live our best life and make the biggest contribution back. And, along the way, it brings you energy, vitality, grace, freedom and love.

"

Do you feel the
desire, the longing, to live
in a different way?
To live with ease and
spaciousness. To stop
punishing yourself or
shaming yourself. And if you
do, that gives you a choice.

"

Body fat

WHERE DOES YOUR BODY FAT LIVE AND WHY?

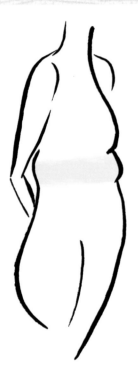

LIVER

FAT DEPOSITION PATTERN:
Liver roll; a roll of fat underneath the bra-line, cellulite.

Needs

- Decrease liver-loaders
  - alcohol
  - trans fats
  - refined and artificial sugars
  - synthetic substances, such as pesticides and non-essential medication, like those found in skin products.
- Increase bitter foods, such as leafy green vegies. Those in the Brassica genus are particularly excellent — broccoli sprouts rock!
- Start the day with lemon juice in warm water.
- No processed foods — this results in lower levels of sugars, inflammatory fats and artificial substances, such as preservatives.
- Resolve any digestion problems, such as diarrhoea, constipation, bloating, irritable bowel syndrome-like symptoms.
- Add to your diet bitter herbs that support bile production and liver detoxification pathways, such as:

  - globe artichoke
  - St Mary's thistle
  - turmeric.

ADRENALS

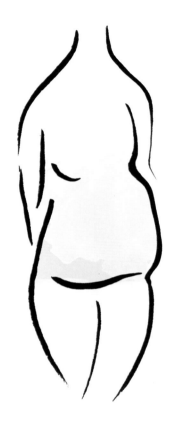

FAT DEPOSITION PATTERN:

Thickening of torso to protect vital organs as the body perceives that the food supply is in danger - the tummy and 'back verandah'

Needs

- Decrease caffeine consumption.
- Explore your perception of pressure and urgency, and save it for when you really need it — not your everyday life.
- Live life in touch with how privileged it is that all of your basic needs are met, whereas for too many people in the world, this is not the case.
- Spend more time diaphragmatically breathing to activate the parasympathetic nervous system (PNS); nothing lowers stress hormones faster than long, slow breaths.
- Remember the serenity prayer: *"Grant me the serenity to accept the things I cannot change, Courage to change the things I can, And wisdom to know the difference."*
- Ensure your diet addresses adrenal support or includes calming nutrients and herbs, depending on the stage of stress.

These nutrients and herbs might include:

- magnesium
- vitamin C
- B vitamins
- withania
- skullcap
- rhodiola
- Siberian ginseng
- licorice
- rehmannia.

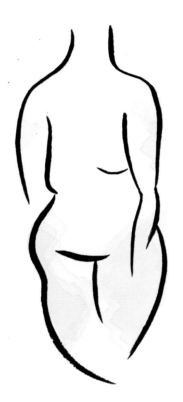

INSULIN

FAT DEPOSITION PATTERN

Starts at belly, then continues all over if blood glucose and insulin levels are not corrected/managed

Needs

- Adopt a low-carbohydrate (sugars and starches) way of eating; remember many alcoholic drinks contain high levels of sugars.
- Avoid processed foods.
- Have small serves of carbs from wholefood sources only, such as sweet potato, pumpkin and brown rice.
- Eat plenty of water-based vegies.
- Exercise daily — walking, strength training, yoga, restorative practices.
- Manage stress and support your adrenals, as living in a state where the sympathetic nervous system (SNS) is dominant leads to the primary utilization of glucose as a fuel (as opposed to body fat), requiring more insulin, which needs to be minimized.
- Some plant medicine along with the aforementioned lifestyle changes can also be useful, such as:

  - bergamot
  - citrus peel extract
  - rehmannia.

ESTROGEN DOMINANCE

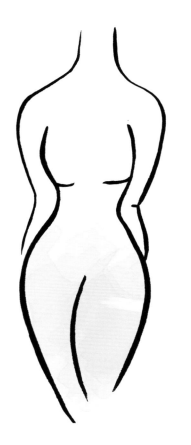

This is often due to liver congestion leading to the recycling of estrogen.

FAT DEPOSITION PATTERN:

Bottom, hips, thighs; pear shape is enhanced; mostly fat below the waist

Needs

- Focus on liver solutions.
- Often stress management and adrenal support are required, as the excessive, relentless output of stress hormones leads to poor progesterone production, which adds to the estrogen dominance.

- Nutrients and herbal medicines that can be beneficial (and don't forget those listed in the liver and adrenal section, as well) include:

  - broccoli sprouts
  - iodine
  - selenium
  - vitamin D
  - plants in the Bupleurum genus
  - plants in the Schisandra genus.

Stuck?

WHY CAN'T YOU LOSE WEIGHT EVEN THOUGH YOU DON'T EAT THAT BADLY?

There are nine factors that impact whether your body is getting the message to store fat or burn it.

They are: calories, stress hormones, sex hormones, liver function, gut bacteria, thyroid function, insulin, the nervous system and emotions. Beyond that though, it is important to recognise what you are eating (of course). And when people say to me "I don't eat that badly", I've found what that means is a day that often looks something like the table on the next page.

So that's about 60 teaspoons of sugar for the day, and that's with a real-food dinner! If it had been spaghetti bolognaise for dinner it would have been 80 teaspoons for the day. And that's without any soft drink, most of which have about 10 to 15 teaspoons of sugar per can. I included the real-food dinner so you could see how few sugars real-food has – yes even a dinner with potatoes. So many people ask me if it's okay to eat potatoes. Ditch the processed foods instead. Sure, numerous whole foods, such as fruit, naturally contain sugars. However, what has dramatically changed in the recent past is the enormous over-consumption of concentrated, refined sugars as they are added to so many processed foods. These are the biggest problem.

So when you look at how you eat, are you seeing the sugars 'hidden' in foods?

Where could you make improvements and lower the sugar content of how you eat?

What real-food swaps could you make to replace some processed foods you regularly eat?

	TEASPOONS OF SUGAR	DAILY TOTAL
BREAKFAST	**JUICE** 1 cup, 25g sugar, 5 tsp **CEREAL** 100g, 35g sugar, 7 tsp + 1 cup milk 15g, 3 tsp **YOGHURT** 200g, 25g sugar, 5 tsp **COFFEE WITH MILK** 1 cup, 15g sugar, 3 tsp	23 teaspoons
SNACK	**COFFEE WITH MILK** 1 cup, 15g sugar, 3 tsp **APPLE** 20g sugar, 4 tsp	7 teaspoons
LUNCH	**SANDWICH WITH CHICKEN, SALAD & MAYONNAISE** 25g sugar, 5 tsp **ORANGE** 20g sugar, 4 tsp	9 teaspoons
SNACK	**SMALL CHOCOLATE BAR** 30g sugar, 6 tsp	6 teaspoons
DRINK	**2 GLASSES OF WHITE WINE** 200ml each, 42g sugar, 8 tsp	8 teaspoons
DINNER	**MEAT AND 5 VEGETABLES:** potato, broccoli, cabbage, cauliflower, beans 2.5g sugar, ½ tsp	1/2 teaspoon
DESSERT	**3 SCOOPS ICE CREAM** 33g sugar, 6.5 tsp	6.5 teaspoon

TOTAL SUGAR: 302.5 grams, 60 teaspoons.

Bloating

WHAT'S CAUSING YOURS?

"How can I be so bloated even though I haven't eaten that badly?" Sound familiar? A bloated tummy can be the bane of your life when you don't know what causes it and more importantly, what to do about it. It can be caused by myriad factors. It may or may not come with a change in bowel habits or flatulence, and with or without pain. So let's take a deeper look at what can lead to bloating.

IRRITABLE BOWEL SYNDROME (IBS)

Studies suggest that IBS affects approximately one in five women in many Western countries. I like to say (as with premenstrual syndrome) that it is common, but is not normal. It is not how it is supposed to be. Food is not supposed to bloat us. Typical symptoms of IBS include bloating, diarrhoea, constipation, or intermittent bouts of both diarrhoea and constipation, mucous in the stool, and excessive flatulence. But you don't have to have IBS to experience bloating.

Regardless of your physical size, if you look down and see a bloated stomach, there can be an alarm that screeches inside your head, whether you recognize it or not, that makes you worry about your physical size. It doesn't matter if you have eaten nutritious food that day and exercised, or eaten poorly and done nothing but sit on your bottom, but if you distinctly recall waking that morning with your tummy feeling comfortable and now it looks like you have swallowed a football, then it tends to have an effect. Logic disappears at this point. If you were still thinking logically, you would tell yourself that it is not possible to gain a football's worth of fat in a day and that your tummy is simply bloated, so calm down, things will be fine again in the morning, and that it would be good to get to the bottom of your

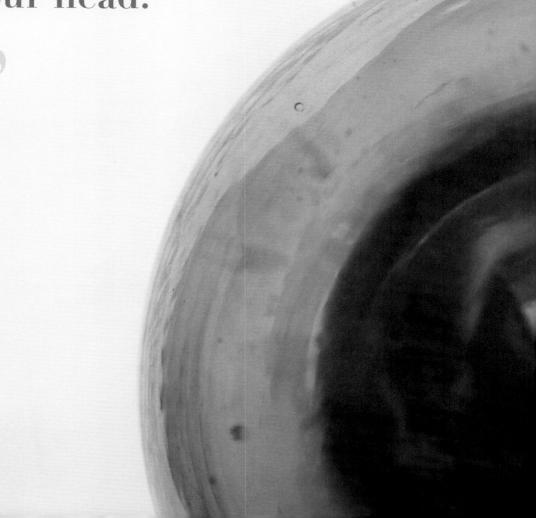

"

If you look down and see a bloated stomach, there can be an alarm that screeches inside your head.

"

bloatedness. But the potential for that logical train tends to leave the station the moment your brain sees your tummy protruding.

Instead, common reactions in the psyche, especially the female one, might be sudden onset of a really bad mood, over-reaction to anything and everything, tears at the drop of a hat, withdrawal, or a major "what the heck" food attack that leaves the pantry bare. Some people are aware of what has led to their change in mood. Most are not. And it is worse for those who have been making massive efforts with food and movement. The people who have eaten poorly that day still feel lousy about themselves, but they follow that lousy feeling with thoughts that drive more even lousy feelings such as, "Well, what did you expect? You ate cake when you said you weren't going to. You're so hopeless, you have no willpower and you'll never change." Really non-uplifting sentiments that do not inspire insights that could lead to a change in behaviour or allow insights to flow!

Such reactions raise numerous issues about beliefs and behaviours, which are explored in *Accidentally Overweight*. However, on a physical level, which is my focus here, it is essential that we examine why your tummy keeps bloating.

- Is it related to your menstrual cycle only?

- Does it only happen after you eat lunch? If so, what are you eating for lunch?

- Does your tummy bloat only after an afternoon snack? What are you choosing to consume at this time of day?

- Is it worse when you are stressed? Did it only begin after you went through a great deal of change, positive or challenging? Did it begin (but perhaps not immediately) after a relationship break-up? Or a period of disordered eating?

- Did it start after an episode of food poisoning, or after a holiday where you had a very upset tummy?

Menstrual cycle-related bloat

If your tummy only bloats in the lead-up to your period, it is likely to be caused by estrogen dominance: too much estrogen (liver-related) or not enough progesterone. Refer to the sex hormone information in this book for steps to take to begin to address this.

After-meal bloating

In my experience working with clients, I have learned that there are some foods that are better eaten on an empty stomach if you have challenges with your digestive system. Fruit is one of them. If bloating is an issue for you, only eat fruit first thing in the morning on an empty stomach — none for lunch and none mid-afternoon. This includes dried fruit. You may find the same thing happens with starchy carbohydrates, such as bread. Some people bloat no matter what time of day they eat bread, and, if that is the case, they will usually do well omitting all gluten-containing grains for a four-week period to see if this is going to make a difference. Others are fine with bread/toast for breakfast, but for lunch it is a disaster in their digestive system. Bread is a highly processed food, after all, with very little nourishment.

All foods containing casein (foods derived from an udder — cow, goat or sheep — although the latter two tend to be tolerated better than cow's milk) can be significant contributors to a bloated stomach. Remove all sources of casein from your diet for a trial period of four weeks, and observe how you feel. Remember, though, that if you omit foods for more than four weeks, it is important you consult an experienced health professional to ensure you are not missing out on specific nutrients.

You will like this next bit even less. Coffee can be incredibly bloating for some people. With a milk-based coffee, it may be the cow's milk or the soy milk, but even black coffee will cause some people to bloat. Biochemically, coffee drives both liver and gallbladder action, plus it triggers the adrenals to secrete adrenalin, which can go on to affect another adrenal hormone, called "aldosterone", one that determines how much fluid your body retains. Switch to herbal tea or green tea, and give coffee a rest for four weeks to see if this solves your bloating. Green tea contains some caffeine (about one-third the caffeine of coffee), but the effects are buffered by another substance in green tea called "theanine". Green tea is also packed with antioxidants and has what are believed to be powerful anti-cancer properties.

Observation is key to this process since your body does not have a voice. Instead, it communicates through symptoms and lets you know when it is happy or not. A food that bloats you is, in that moment, not your friend, and your body is simply letting you know. Do not let your head run away with you when you notice this, though. Remind yourself that just because it bloats you today does not mean you will never eat that food or drink that drink again. It simply means that right now, in this moment, it does not serve you. So take a four-week break from whatever you suspect. No tears, no tantrums, just cut it out for four weeks. You will feel so different when you feed your body precisely what it wants and what nourishes it. Never waste a bloated tummy. Ask it what it wants to tell you, as silly as that may sound. Your body has a wonderful wisdom.

Bloated since a stressful experience

If your tummy changed after a challenging time in your life, it is quite likely that your bloated abdomen was initially due to poor stomach acid production. Now, however, if poor stomach acid production has been ongoing because of an almost low-grade (or high-grade) anxiety inside you, the changes in digestion that were initially caused by poor stomach acid production may have changed the gut bacteria and hence the pH of the large bowel. The first steps here are to stimulate stomach acid using lemon in warm water or apple cider vinegar before meals, and eat in a calm state, as challenging as that may be at times. Restorative practices will be essential for your gut healing and for the digestive system to receive the resources it needs to do its job well.

Adrenal support for stress management may also be needed. Restorative practices (for their calming action on the adrenals and the nervous system), and herbs such as licorice can be immensely beneficial. If bloating began after heartbreak, ask the discomfort what it wants you to know. You may feel a little odd having a conversation with your tummy, but your body knows the truth, and you might be surprised at the message it has for you.

Bloated since food-poisoning episode or upset tummy while travelling

Despite negative stool tests, I have seen this health picture frequently. Where once someone had an iron gut, they now feel like they react to everything. Even if you had forgotten that a gastroenteritis episode began your digestive system challenges, I suggest you do the following:

- discuss having a Helicobacter pylori test with your general practitioner (GP)

- take a herbal anti-parasitic tablet or liquid, even if your stool test came back negative. Be guided by a health professional, but you usually need relatively high doses three times a day, and you need to take them for a two-month period. If a parasite infection is the basis of your ongoing tummy trouble, the natural medicine must be taken for the full two months, as initially only the live parasites are killed by the herbs. As unpleasant as this is to think about, the parasites will have laid eggs in your bowel, and you want the herbs in your gut at the ready, in order to get rid of them immediately as they hatch, if this is the case

- dietary change as outlined above can be very useful in this situation until the gut has healed. What has become known as a "caveman"-style diet (or the Paleolithic or Primal diet; please note, though, there is no one way people from the Paleolithic era ate; in a modern dietary sense, this name refers to a way of eating primarily wholefoods) that is

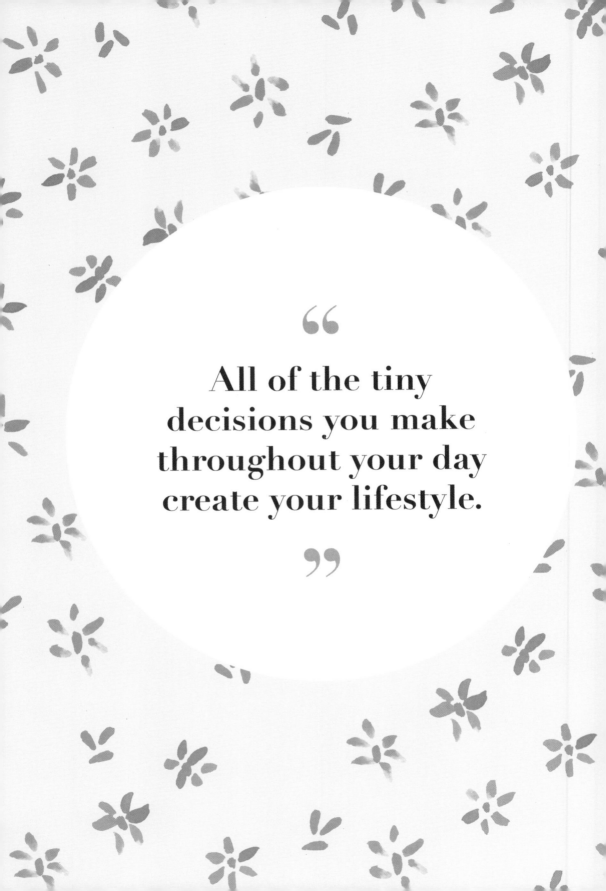

"

All of the tiny decisions you make throughout your day create your lifestyle.

"

both milk- and grain-free can be beneficial. This way of eating also includes broths, which are highly nourishing for the gut. The Specific Carbohydrate Diet (SCD) has also been noted to have excellent results for gut health challenges and to alter gut bacteria profiles

- a low-FODMAPs diet has also been shown to be highly beneficial for people with gut-based health challenges. FODMAPs is an acronym referring to fermentable, oligosaccharides, disaccharides, monosaccharides and polyols. These are complex names for a collection of molecules found in food that are poorly absorbed by some people. When the molecules are poorly absorbed in the small intestine of the digestive tract, these molecules then continue their journey along the digestive tract, arriving at the large intestine, where they act as a food source to the bacteria that live there. The bacteria then digest/ferment these FODMAPs and can cause symptoms of IBS. The fermentation action of gut bacteria on FODMAPs can also be one reason why some people feel better without fruit (or with only small amounts of specific fruits) when they have gut or autoimmune symptoms.

The 3pm slump

It's 3pm. You are at your desk at work and you can barely keep your eyes open. The day seems like it has come to a complete halt. *When will it be hometime? Ahh maybe I need something sweet, or maybe I just need a coffee… Yes!! That's it — that will give me energy. But I also need something sweet… Maybe there's still some of that chocolate cake left over from the morning tea we had earlier. Yes, that's it, I'll have coffee and cake, then I'll be awake. And then I'll be able to make it through the rest of my day.*

Sound familiar? Many people feel an energy slump at 3pm, which is typically followed by food or beverage choices to remedy this — typically those that are high in sugar or don't serve their health in any way. Many people describe it as though something else takes control of their decision making — someone else takes over their body. As they try every strategy to get through "the afternoon slump", where typically they have no energy, they turn to sugar and refined carbohydrates, in a desperate attempt to boost their flagging energy.

A combination of stress hormones, caffeine and a blood sugar roller-coaster is often to blame in this situation. Adrenalin, one of our stress hormones, is produced when we perceive that there is pressure and/or urgency, or when we consume caffeine. The production of adrenalin triggers the release of glucose into the blood, to help fuel us to get away from the supposed danger we are in. However, for many people today, their stress is perceived — they are not in fact being chased — so this glucose goes unused and is then stored as fat, thanks to insulin.

This whole process can leave us feeling tired and reaching for the closest carbohydrate-laden food to satisfy the craving for the sugars we have just used up. This can happen throughout the day,

and causes highs and lows in blood glucose levels. With a view to preventing that craving for sugar in the afternoon, the first step is to take a break from the daily coffee, and replace it with herbal tea. Sorry! But it's game-changing in resolving sugar cravings for many people.

Food solutions

The more you train your body to utilize body fat as a preferential fuel source efficiently (instead of glucose), the less hungry you will be. This is impacted on by the stress response, as well as by what you eat. Eating fat is critical, fat from wholefood sources, such as avocado, nuts, seeds, coconut, organic butter, sustainable, wild-caught oily fish and pasture-fed meats, while at the same time omitting refined sugars. Get your sugars from vegetables, fruit (two pieces per day suits most people), legumes and pulses.

A good breakfast in the morning containing real-food fat will help to satisfy and fuel you through the morning. Manage stress using your breath, for example, and refuel with real-food choices throughout the day to ensure you maintain even blood glucose levels, rather than let your blood glucose level fall too low, requiring adrenalin to be made to increase it. When your body becomes more efficient at utilizing body fat as a fuel, it means better and more consistent energy and mood — plus your clothes fit you better. Not to mention that you generate fewer substances that speed up the aging and degeneration process.

Many people find that they are less likely to reach for sweet food in the afternoon if they have a source of wholefood fat at lunchtime, in particular. Try adding some of the suggestions above to lunch, or take pre-prepared subtly sweet snacks that are also rich in wholefood fats to have on hand at 3pm. Brain balls are a great example: a snack made of a few dates, nuts, seeds and a little bit of cacao powder.

Non-food solutions

Aside from food and preventing the crash in the first place, here are three ways to lift your energy at 3pm.

Have a cup of green tea instead of coffee

1 Green tea is a wonderfully uplifting beverage to consume. It contains a small amount of caffeine, as well as an amino acid called "l-theanine", which boosts energy levels but also helps to keep us calm. Packed full of antioxidants, it is a health-promoting alternative to coffee. If you are highly caffeine-sensitive, have a refreshing mint tea instead, as you don't want the caffeine to interfere with your sleep.

Close open tabs at work

Work on closing what I call "open tabs" — tasks, emails or jobs that haven't been resolved. We walk around each day with so many "tabs" open — like websites sitting open on your computer screen — that it is little wonder we feel drained or flattened. Schedule tasks instead of just listing them. (See details of this elsewhere in the book.) **2**

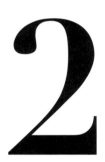

Go for a walk

3 It might seem like a paradox — and often the last thing you might feel like doing — but a brisk walk is one of the best ways to naturally boost your energy. It is great for circulation, increases oxygen supply to the cells of your body, and helps you feel more alert. It's a wonderful way to break up your day, too: try going for a walk around 3pm, which is often the time people start to crave sugar.

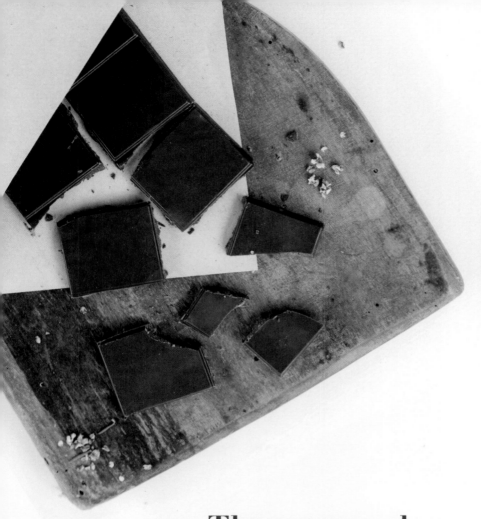

There are only two fuels
for the human body: glucose
and fat. And when you are
living on stress hormones
your body predominantly
uses glucose as its fuel,
not body fat.

Craving sugar

WHY YOU MIGHT FIND IT HARD TO RESIST

Many people today know they need to eat less sugar or cut it out of their diet completely. You would have to have had your head buried in the sand not to know that eating refined sugars does not serve your health in any way. Yet, even with great understanding of this topic and even with the desire to change dietary sugar habits, many people describe it as being the major challenge for them on their road to outstanding health. So why is it that we crave sugar so much?

One reason is certainly habit. Another is its infiltration into the food supply, even into savoury-tasting foods, and a taste preference for sweeter and sweeter foods is also playing a role. It is a case of more begets more. Very few people go back after dinner for a second helping of broccoli. Yet what most people are not familiar with is the impact of the biochemistry — of stress hormone production — on sugar cravings.

As you now understand, there are only two fuels for the human body: glucose and fat. And when you are living on stress hormones because of too much caffeine or due to your perception of pressure and urgency, your body predominantly uses glucose as its fuel, not body fat.

A person weighing 70 kilograms has the capacity to store about 2,500 calories of glucose (as glycogen in their liver and muscles), while that same person will store about 130,000 calories of fat. So the more your body thinks it needs to use glucose as your fuel to help you escape from danger, the more it needs to keep your "get out of danger" fuel-tank full. So you crave it to support yet another survival mechanism.

Too many people in the Western world today regularly over-consume caffeine, feel pressured about their work, money, relationships or their body, and feel like all of their tasks are urgent, like there aren't enough hours in the day, and they scratch the itch of their "not enoughness" (see my TEDx talk for more about this, as well as the section about it later in this book) on and off all day. Then they crave wine in the evenings for the sugar and to help them relax, even though underneath they are utterly exhausted. And many people have become so accustomed to living this way that they don't even notice how stressed they are anymore. Anxiety is rife, yet most people who experience it have not been informed that caffeine leads them to make the very hormone that drives anxious feelings. If you experience such feelings, caffeine needs to be the first thing that goes.

When you live like this, your body will predominantly use glucose as a fuel in preference to body fat, and it will only switch back to being an efficient fat-burner if you make some changes. You can start with the food — some people do — yet for others starting here is precisely why they have made no progress in decreasing or cutting out refined sugars and refined starches. (Both sugars and starches are broken down to glucose in the digestive system.)

So if you know that starting with food is not your way, then park it. You can start by focusing on activating your parasympathetic nervous system (PNS), which means embracing diaphragmatic breathing. This may take the form of a restorative, breath-focused practice, such as restorative yoga, t'ai chi, meditation, or simply taking regular intervals across the day where you commit to 20 long, slow breaths that move your belly as you breathe. It is a matter of

The calmer you feel, the more your PNS is activated, and the less sugar your body will need to keep the glucose fuel-tank full.

retraining yourself to breathe this way, instead of the short, sharp, shallow breaths in your upper chest that adrenalin drives. The calmer you feel, the more your PNS is activated, and the less sugar your body will need to keep the glucose fuel-tank full.

Increasing your intake of green vegetables and/or dietary fats from wholefood sources can also make a big difference in reducing your desire for sugar. A high intake of green leafy vegetables for a minimum of 21 days starts to change your taste preferences, as greens have a bitter taste base. When it comes to fat, if you have lived through the "low fat, high carb" era and you became conscious of your dietary fat intake, you may not be eating enough of it. Notice when you crave sugar, and significantly increase your intake of fats at the meal prior to the typical craving time. For example, if the middle of the afternoon is your tough time, then eat more wholefood fat at lunchtime.

Fat is incredibly satiating, and you'll notice it will fuel you for longer through your afternoon. Yet if you still have the mindset that counting calories is your only road to weight loss, you'll never let yourself eat the fat, given it has the highest number of calories per gram. However, when you eat carbohydrates it leads the body to make insulin, which you now understand signals to the body to store fat, whereas when you eat dietary fat, no fat-storage signalling hormones are released. Not all calories behave equally inside the body, a concept I explore in detail in my book *The Calorie Fallacy*.

If you crave sugar, you might like to try some of the following tips to help break this pattern:

- eat more wholefood fat at the meal before you crave sugar. For example, if 3pm is your tough time, then amp up the fat at lunchtime. If it is after dinner, then increase the fat particularly at dinner

- have subtly sweet food on hand that serves your health for the time you know the cravings set in. Take some time on a Sunday and pre-prepare a batch of brain balls, for example, so you have a snack ready to go that satisfies the desire for sweetness on the taste buds but is rich in wholefood fats. This means you don't need to eat many of them to be satisfied

- amp up your greens! Bitter-tasting foods, such as green vegies, help quell our desire for and enjoyment of excessive amounts of sweet food. Try adding to your day an organic green drink powder, made up of ground-up vegetables, so you get a concentrated nutritional boost plus the flow-on effects of the greens

- decrease adrenalin production, so your body feels "safe" to use body fat as a fuel. This means getting honest with yourself about how much caffeine you are having. Some people do really well just cutting back, while others need to omit it for four to 12 weeks. To decrease adrenalin production, you will also need to explore your perception of pressure and urgency, and save it for when you really need it; don't make what you need to do each day be full of pressure and urgency

- activate the PNS by embracing long, slow diaphragmatic breaths.

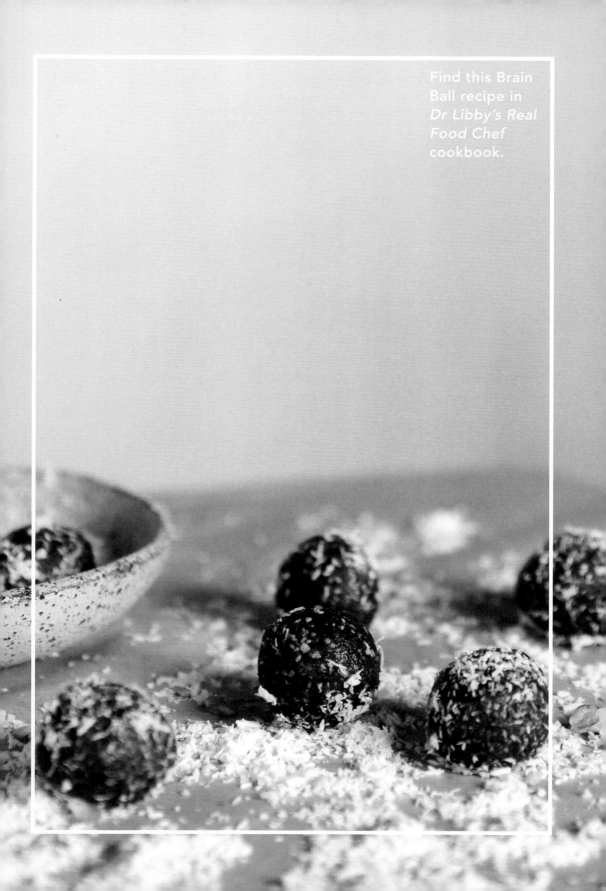

Find this Brain
Ball recipe in
*Dr Libby's Real
Food Chef*
cookbook.

Lifestyle and rituals

CREATE A GOOD MORNING

What you do to begin your day can enhance or hinder your quality of life, including your health, in a major way. There are rituals we can embrace so easily, yet they are also easy not to do. Take brushing your teeth, for example. It doesn't take long, it's easy to do, but it would also be just as easy not to do it. Yet when you think about the long-term trajectory your life would take if you didn't brush your teeth each day, the consequences range from necessary expensive dental work to malnutrition due to not being able to chew your food properly. In other words, when we don't do these little things, it can affect the quality of our lives, as well as what we get to experience today.

Creating a morning ritual is one of the most beneficial undertakings you can do. When you open your eyes to greet a new day, you might decide to think of five things for which you are grateful, before you arise. You might get up and scrape your tongue, drink a glass of water and meditate. You might go for a walk or go to the gym, write in a journal, read, or gaze out the window at your surroundings, grateful for your freedom or considering how you could contribute even more to this world. Regardless of what you do, this non-negotiable morning ritual sets you up for the day, physically, mentally, emotionally and/or spiritually.

Meeting the needs of young children doesn't need to interfere with a morning ritual — no matter how big or small — that can foster immense spaciousness across your day. Do what you can. If your morning ritual involves the need for solitude, for example, you might decide to get up 20 minutes before everyone else in the household. Or welcome the opportunity to teach children (albeit not very young ones, of course) to occupy themselves while you do your thing. Another key, however, is that we all need to remain flexible so that if a child needs us during this time, it doesn't "ruin" the morning. It just is what it is. And there's immense beauty in that, too.

When you set up your day and get plugged into your natural, inner intelligence, you are in the right relationship with yourself, which allows you to be true to others. Plus, you get more done. You also have healthier interactions, and, given that poor-quality interactions are one of the major sources of stress for many people today, this counts. When you set up your day, your mind is sharp, you hold your body more strongly, and you are more effective in your workday. You cope better with whatever comes your way. People I have worked with who have embraced a morning ritual have also suggested that they are better colleagues, parents, partners and friends when they have set up their day. So the ripple effect of a morning ritual is significant. Not only do you tend to experience better and more consistent energy, but those around you get the best version of you, too.

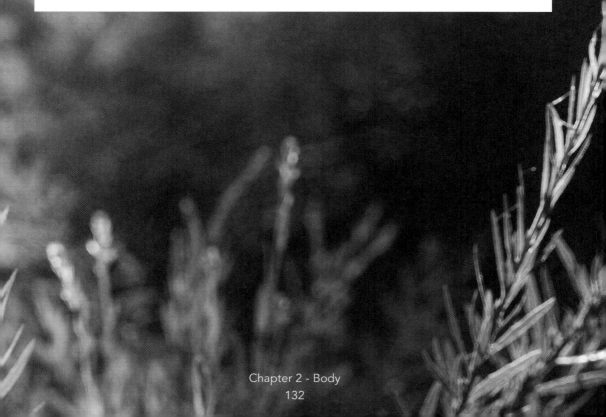

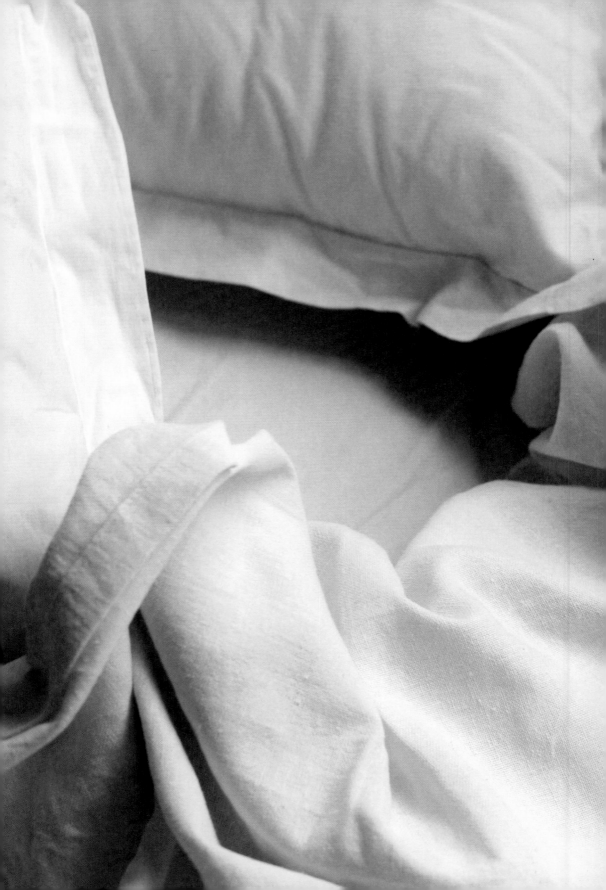

Sleep

WHY GOOD SLEEP MATTERS

Sleep is a topic I feel incredibly passionate about for a huge number of reasons. When we are exhausted, everything in life feels more difficult. So I want to give you very practical information, things you can actually apply to your life to make a really big difference in this area. Before we discuss what to do about sleep that is not restorative, it is first important for you to understand why sleep can become disrupted and ineffective in its purpose of rest, repair and restoration. I also want to show you how common it is now to sleep poorly — common, but not normal, as I like to say.

In February 2013, my team and I conducted a survey asking people who read our Facebook page (*facebook.com/DrLibbyLive*) about their sleep. Over 500 people answered our questions. Of those, 97 per cent shared with us that they wake up feeling tired. Only 3 per cent of people reported waking up with energy.* Think about that. Waking unrefreshed is a really big deal. Furthermore, the majority of people who responded couldn't sleep through the night either, and this is an area that, once it is optimal, will make a significant difference to so many aspects of your health and beauty. As I said, everything feels more difficult when we are exhausted, so let's get you sleeping restoratively.

* Please note that this is not scientific research, but a survey. One could argue that people who are drawn to learn more about their body and/or who have challenges with sleep may be more likely to comment on a sleep survey. I am simply pointing out that large numbers of people don't sleep restoratively.

Sleep, and the rest and repair it offers our body, is critical to life. With great sleep, we have improved memory and cognition, and better immune function. Sometimes when I talk about immune function, I sense that the importance of this system doesn't fully register with some people. Many people simply link great immune function with minimizing how many colds and bouts of flu they get. Yet your immune function is critical in the prevention of cancer, as well as in the prevention of autoimmune diseases, such as multiple sclerosis, lupus and coeliac disease, all of which are on the rise. Taking great care of our immune system is of immense importance to our long-term health and quality of life, and sleep plays an enormous role in whether our immune system is able to function appropriately or not.

With restorative sleep, we have improved mood, enhanced physical and emotional resilience, increased physical endurance and better hormonal function. When our sleep cycles are disrupted, both our stress hormones and our sex hormone balances can be impacted, too.

Everything works better with restorative sleep: our digestive system, our sex hormone balance, our mood, our skin and even our thyroid function. A recent clinical trial found that sleep quality impacts skin function and aging. If you have poor sleep quality or do not get enough sleep, your skin finds it harder to recover from free radical damage, such as sun exposure and environmental toxins.

I wanted to open this section by showing you just how far-reaching amazing sleep can be, because you may just think "Oh, I wake up tired most of the time, but isn't that normal?" No, it is common, but it is not normal. Many people blame age for why they start to feel more and more tired as the years go by, but it doesn't have to be this way. If low energy truly was down to age, then every 82-year-old I know would be exhausted, and they're not! We can make a really big difference to how we feel and function, both on the inside and the outside, through good-quality sleep.

Sleep required

How much sleep do you actually need? Our requirements vary based on our gender, our age and our physical demands. There are studies that suggest that adults have a very basic sleep requirement of seven to eight hours per night. Other compelling studies show eight to eight-and-a-half hours per night is actually critical for all of the vital repair work that has to go on inside your body while you are asleep.

We are essentially the health of our cells, and cellular repair takes place during sleep. Everything from skin cells to the cells that make up our muscles need repair work overnight. When cells are working optimally, we look and feel our best. I want to remind you that we cannot fight our biology: our biology is our biology, and we need eight hours of sleep a night. When we are not getting that, all sorts of bodily functions can be disrupted.
So, let's help you achieve blissful sleep!

Sleep requirements tend to be based somewhat on our age. Newborn babies need a lot of sleep; although many of you may have experienced first-hand that some babies need more than others. Some like or need a lot of sleep, perhaps 18 hours a day, and then there are those who need somewhat less, perhaps 12 or 14 hours a day. Infants, toddlers and preschoolers need less sleep than newborns, but still substantially more than teenagers. Sleep needs continue to gradually decline, and by the time children are teenagers they need between about eight-and-a-half and nine-and-a-quarter hours per night. I have deep concerns, however, over what's happening for our teenagers, because many of them are taking back-lit devices to bed, such as iPads, laptops and cellphones. And the light that is emitted from these devices can significantly disrupt the production of the sleep hormone called "melatonin". Light destroys melatonin, as you will learn more about in a moment, which is one reason why I have deep concerns for teens who may not be getting enough hours of sleep to do the vital growth and repair work that needs to happen. As mentioned above, an adult's biological requirement for sleep is essentially seven to nine hours of sleep per night.

Sleep as a priority

For many people, to improve their sleep it needs to become a priority. So many people today compromise their sleep to get more done in a day. They wake up earlier and go to bed later in an attempt to get more tasks done. Yet when you deeply appreciate how non-negotiable sleep is for your health, you make it a priority.

What interferes with restorative sleep?

When sleeping pills are used as a bridge, as a short-term band-aid for sleep problems, there is potentially no problem. But until the deeper issue(s) that created the sleep issue in the first place are addressed, no progress will be made to allow the person to come off the sleeping pills and begin sleeping naturally again. So people come to rely on medication for their sleep, and it is this long-term use that I am concerned about. The deeper issue(s) must be addressed or other health challenges can potentially arise. I call it "getting to the heart of the matter". And sometimes the heart of the matter is physical (biochemical), such as too much caffeine or alcohol, and sometimes it is emotional. For example, you may lie awake at night worrying that you let someone down that day.

Another great thing to ask yourself is when the last time was that you slept well. If it was when you were on holiday, you can bet that stress is playing a big role in your not sleeping well in your usual life. If the last time you slept well was in a hotel, again it may be worthwhile to consider how stress may be involved, but also look at what you are sleeping on. People often keep their beds for far too long; in a hotel, the beds tend to be newer, so it might simply be the structural support that you were getting in a hotel that allowed you to rest easy. Pay attention to whether you sleep better when you have a small meal for dinner, or even for some reason skip dinner. You may like to try omitting spicy food in the evening, or eating smaller portions, as this may positively impact on your sleep.

"

It is what you
do every day that
impacts on your
health, not what you
do occasionally.

"

Maybe the last time you slept well was after abstaining from alcohol. The reality is that alcohol disrupts rapid eye movement (REM) sleep, the fourth part of our sleep cycle, during which time the critical repair work is done inside our body. Even though alcohol tends to make people fall asleep quite quickly, it can disrupt our sleep cycles, as it interferes with REM sleep. Notice how alcohol consumption affects your sleep, and consider making changes.

The last time you slept well may have been before you had children. If you sleep quite well but your sleep is interrupted because little ones need you in the night, please remember that they are young for such a short period of time, and there will come a time when they will sleep through the night. Worrying about your sleep, and the disruptions that you can't do anything about, only serves to disrupt your sleep further. So I encourage you to accept that right now your sleep will be disrupted, and make the most of the nights when it is not!

Your sleep

How many hours a night (on average)
do you currently sleep for?

How many hours a night would
you like to sleep for?

If those two numbers above are not the same, what insight
have you received that could change this for you?

Why we have big conversations at night,

NOT AT BREAKFAST

Melatonin is your primary sleep hormone; it helps you fall asleep and stay asleep. However, its production in your body is interfered with by light. Relatively speaking, it wasn't too long ago that we rose with the sun and rested soon after sundown. Obviously that all changed with the invention of electricity.

When you expose your eyes to light too late into the evening, through any means, including the use of back-lit devices, such as iPads, mobile phones and laptops, or you work until late under bright light, or watch television, it can stop your body from producing the very hormone that is necessary for great sleep. If you don't wake up refreshed, or particularly if you have trouble falling asleep, become very aware of how much light you are exposing your eyes to within two hours of bedtime. If sleep is a challenge for you, do what you can to only be in soft light in the lead-up to bedtime, and make your bedroom a television-and wireless-device-free zone.

Another powerful way to help reset your body's own natural circadian rhythm is to get up at the same time each morning and expose your eyes to light. Preferably get up and go outside and exercise. If that is not practical for you — perhaps because you have young children who need you — then, on waking, get up and fling the curtains open and notice the day and Nature outside; think of three or five things you are grateful for, and allow your eyes to gently be exposed to the light of this new day. Commit to doing this for a week minimum, and begin to notice the difference.

Chapter 2 - Body
142

Melatonin has an antagonistic relationship with serotonin, one of our happy, calm, content hormones. Antagonistic means that both substances can't be elevated at the same time. When one is high, the other tends to be low. Your circadian rhythm guides serotonin to be high during the day, helping you to feel good, and melatonin is designed to be high through the night, supporting your sleep.

The serotonin–melatonin seesaw, as I have come to call it, is I think one of the reasons why couples tend to have big conversations in the evening. Up until late afternoon, you may have been going along just fine, content, regardless of what was or wasn't going on in your life. Your serotonin level is still okay, and you aren't focused on anything you want. Then, if serotonin levels plummet instead of gradually falling away, you may start to feel like you want something, but you don't know what it is.

Whenever you ask your brain a question, it always comes up with an answer, so be very aware of the quality of questions you ask yourself! Perhaps you say, "I feel like I want something. I'm not sure what it is, but I want something. A minute ago I felt fine, and now I feel like I've got an itch I can't scratch and I want something. What do I want?!"
If big things such as "I want... to move house" or "I want... to renovate the bathroom yesterday" or "I want... to have a baby" don't surface, you will still be feeling like you want something, and you might decide it must be food that you want. So you will open the door of the pantry and stand there looking inside, as if the meaning of life is in that cupboard! You get what I mean.

Whenever you ask your brain a question, it always comes up with an answer, so be very aware of the quality of questions you ask yourself!

Humans instinctively know that carbohydrate-rich foods promote serotonin production, which is partly why when the "I want something" syndrome hits you might head for the pantry. We hope that what we want is in there. Usually guilt is all we find.

The morning time can also prove to be a challenge for someone in this pattern, as serotonin can be slow to rise. As you now know, melatonin is destroyed by sunlight, which is partly why when we go outside and exercise in the morning we feel so great all day. The melatonin plummets when the retina of our eyes is exposed to light and, as a result, our serotonin surges. On a day with that hormonal profile, we can cope with just about anything. The flip-side, though, is not so appealing. If we have gone to bed after midnight, not slept well, and have children or work to get up for, or all of these factors, we may not want to rise with the sun, as we don't feel rested. If we don't have early-morning commitments and just wander out of bed at some point during the morning, our melatonin slowly seeps away, and our serotonin slowly rises. On a day like this, we feel like we need a few coffees to get us going.

If this tale is ringing true for you, and the carb-fest in the evening feels out of control, the solution may not initially be dietary in nature, as fighting the carb cravings can feel hugely challenging when this is going on. Step one is to start getting up at the same time each morning and going outside and moving. Or at least open the curtains and recognize that a new day has dawned. Welcome the day with t'ai chi, a walk, yoga — whatever feels right to your body. Commit to doing this for four weeks, every day. Yes, every day. Your sleep, your serotonin and that itch of wanting something that is never satisfied in the evening will love you for it.

Liver love

When it comes to every aspect of our health, the liver packs a mighty punch. It is one of the big guns when it comes to your energy, vitality and hormonal balance, as well as to the clarity of your skin and eyes. In conjunction with the gallbladder, the liver works endlessly to help us excrete fatty substances that the body no longer needs, including old hormones, pesticides and stored body fat.

The liver is the body's second largest organ after our skin. It sits behind your right ribcage. Its primary role is detoxification, a concept that has had much confusion surrounding it — confusion we are about to resolve.

A simple way to imagine the detoxification power of the liver is to picture a triangle shape: inside that triangle are billions and billions of little circles, each one of them a liver cell. Imagine that inside each liver cell is a wheel spinning. Each turn of the wheel drives your liver function.

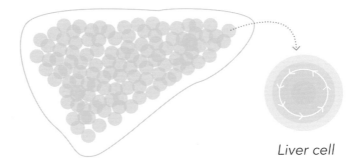

Liver cell

When we treat our liver unkindly, a circle can die, and for a time the liver can regenerate a new cell to replace the dead cell, but after a while this is no longer possible, and a globule of fat can take up residence where once that fat-burning, detoxification wheel was working.

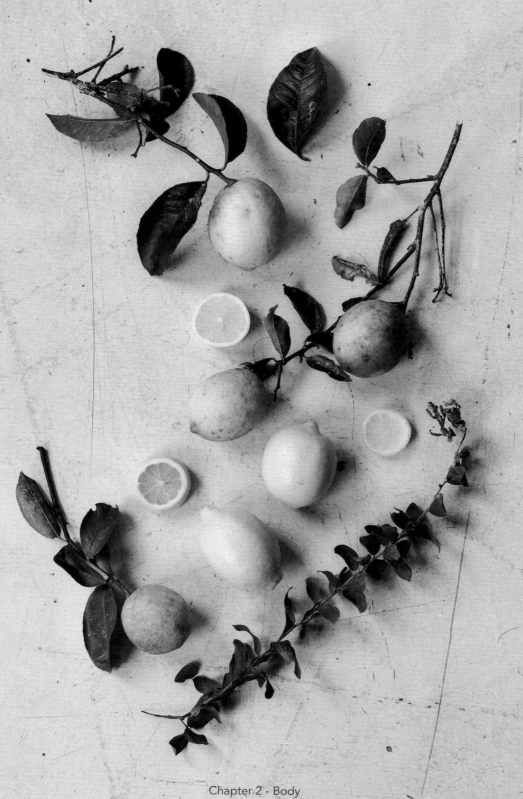

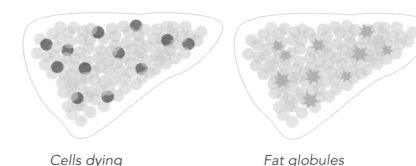

Cells dying   *Fat globules*

When many fat globules take over (known as "fatty liver"), health can suffer significantly. Less efficient detoxification processes can lead to poor thyroid function, sex hormone imbalances, congested skin, lousy cholesterol levels, and impaired blood glucose management that often shows up as sugar cravings. Moreover, where our body wants to lay down body fat can also shift. For the first time people may notice that they have a fat roll quite high up on their abdomen, which is called a "liver roll". For women this is just below their bra-line, and for men, just beneath their pectoral muscles.

In the not-too-distant past, only people who regularly over-consumed alcohol developed fatty liver disease, but now we are seeing teenagers develop it simply from eating diets high in processed foods and drinks. This has become so common that a new disease has been named, called "non-alcoholic fatty liver disease". Imagine a liver that looks just like one that has been chronically battered by alcohol, yet processed food has created it.

DETOXIFICATION

The mechanisms of detoxification and elimination that your body utilizes are critical to understand in creating any optimal health plan, as, when they are compromised, every process inside of us that creates health will be affected. This is particularly true for sex hormone balance, whether we burn body fat or store it, as well as the body's ability to prevent major diseases.

There are numerous organs and body systems involved in detoxification. They include:

- the liver transforms substances that if they were to accumulate, they would harm you, altering them into less harmful substances you can then excrete

- the colon (digestive system) contains bacteria that produce both healthy and unhealthy substances, so you want to keep your bowel moving regularly, as one of its roles is to release waste and problematic substances so that they do not accumulate

- the kidneys are constantly filtering your blood and getting rid of anything you don't need, including toxins, via urine

- the skin not only protects and houses your organs, but it allows problematic substances to leave the body via perspiration

- the respiratory system plays a key role in the detoxification squad — even the hairs inside your nose help filter the air you breathe in — while the lungs are responsible for filtering out fumes, allergens, mould and airborne toxins; when we are stressed, we tend to shift from slow belly-breathing to short, shallow upper-chest breaths, which in turn can reduce the lungs' ability to transport oxygen to all of our tissues; for those of you who know my work, you now know another reason (other than the nervous system and stress-hormone lowering benefits) why diaphragmatic breathing is my number one health tip.

Detoxification is a process that goes on inside us all day, every day. The choices we make influence how efficiently the liver is able to do its job. Detoxification is essentially a transformation process. Any substance that would be harmful to you if it accumulated in your body must be changed into a less harmful form so that it can then be excreted safely from your body. To look and feel your best, you want this to be a highly efficient process.

There are two stages to the detoxification process, appropriately named phase 1 and phase 2 liver detoxification. Both phases require certain nutrients to function, and dietary choices can influence how efficiently each phase is able to work. The figure below illustrates the phases of detoxification, and you can see some of the nutrients that are required.

DETOXIFICATION PATHWAYS IN THE LIVER

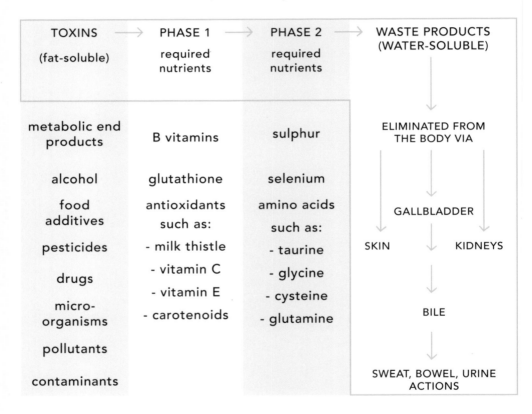

TOXINS (fat-soluble)	PHASE 1 required nutrients	PHASE 2 required nutrients	WASTE PRODUCTS (WATER-SOLUBLE)
metabolic end products	B vitamins	sulphur	ELIMINATED FROM THE BODY VIA
alcohol	glutathione	selenium	
food additives	antioxidants such as:	amino acids such as:	GALLBLADDER
pesticides	- milk thistle	- taurine	SKIN KIDNEYS
drugs	- vitamin C	- glycine	
	- vitamin E	- cysteine	
micro-organisms	- carotenoids	- glutamine	BILE
pollutants			
contaminants			SWEAT, BOWEL, URINE ACTIONS

PHASE 1

For the first stage of detoxification, numerous nutrients, including B vitamins, are essential. Wholegrains are one of the richest sources of B vitamins we have in the food supply; however, many people feel much better with fewer or none of these foods in their diets. People decrease or cut grains out of their diets for various reasons. Some first experienced rapid weight loss with the advent of the high-protein, very low-carbohydrate diets, purported as the ultimate answer to weight-loss desires in the late 1990s, a repeat of the popular dietary concept from the 1970s, and a natural progression from the high-carbohydrate, low-fat guidelines that had preceded them. Others simply started to notice that foods made from grains induced reflux or made their tummy bloated, and they took action to change how they felt. If grains feel good for you and energize you, then enjoy them in wholefood form; some are best soaked prior to consumption. If they don't suit you, don't eat them. Your body knows best what works for you. Simply be aware that if you have a low intake of B vitamins, your phase 1 liver detoxification processes may not function optimally. It can be useful to take a supplement if you eat a low-carbohydrate diet or avoid/limit grains.

PHASE 2

There is one road into the liver, and five (or we could argue six) pathways out of the liver. Just as for phase 1 reactions, phase 2 liver pathways also require certain nutrients to function, in particular, specific amino acids and sulphur.

We get our amino acids from protein foods. Think about this next statement: what we eat becomes a part of us. Protein foods are broken down into amino acids, and they go on to create all of the cells of your immune system, which are what defends you from infection. Amino acids also go on to create the neurotransmitters in your brain that influence your mood and your clarity of thought. They also build your pretty muscles that allow you to carry your groceries. What you eat really does matter — your food becomes a part of you.

For further phase 2 support we need sulphur, which we obtain from eggs, onion, garlic and shallots, as well as from the Brassica genus of vegetables, which includes broccoli, cabbage, kale, Brussels sprouts and cauliflower. The liver makes enzymes that are responsible for the transformation of each substance, and the rate of production of these essential enzymes determines how quickly each substance is processed. The load placed on the liver also determines how quickly things move through the liver, and you will see shortly how all of this impacts on how you look and feel, as well as how your clothes fit you. I believe it is one of the biggest reasons why the calorie equation is redundant in today's world.

LIVER-LOADERS

There is a group of substances I lovingly label "liver-loaders".

They include:

- alcohol
- caffeine
- trans fats
- refined sugars
- synthetic substances, such as pesticides, medications, skincare products
- infections; for example, viruses such as glandular fever (also known as Epstein–Barr virus, mononucleosis).

It is important to do what we can to minimize our exposure to, and consumption of, pesticides and herbicides. Firstly, a number of these synthetic chemicals mimic estrogen and can bind to the estrogen receptors in the body, which has consequences for males and females of all ages. Another concern with the consumption of pesticides and herbicides is the risk of their storage in the fatty tissue of our body. We don't know the long-term consequences of this, or of being exposed to these substances for an entire lifetime, as we are essentially the first generation of people to be exposed to some of them for such a long period. Do we yet know the extent of their cumulative impact on metabolism, let alone other aspects of our health?

ARE YOU CAUGHT IN THIS VICIOUS CYCLE?

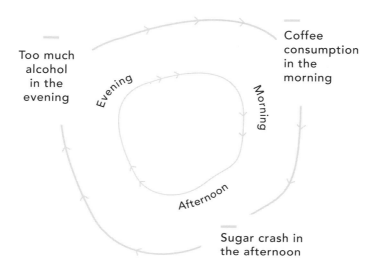

Too much alcohol in the evening

Coffee consumption in the morning

Evening

Morning

Afternoon

Sugar crash in the afternoon

INTERNAL SUBSTANCES REQUIRING DETOXIFICATION

However, it is not just infections or the things we consume or put on our skin that can place demands on the detoxification processes of the liver. Substances your body makes itself also need transformation by the liver so that they can be excreted.

These substances include:

- cholesterol
- steroid (sex) hormones, such as estrogen
- substances created by, or causing, any short-fall in digestion, due to compromised digestive processes
- untreated food sensitivities
- undiagnosed coeliac disease.

I have met countless people who have not consumed much in the way of liver-loaders, but have diabolical menstrual cycles or an ongoing challenge with irritable bowel syndrome or constipation, and often exhibit what I consider to be distinct signs that their liver needs support. Passing clots while menstruating is a classic sign of liver congestion, as are many skin conditions. More symptoms are listed on the following pages.

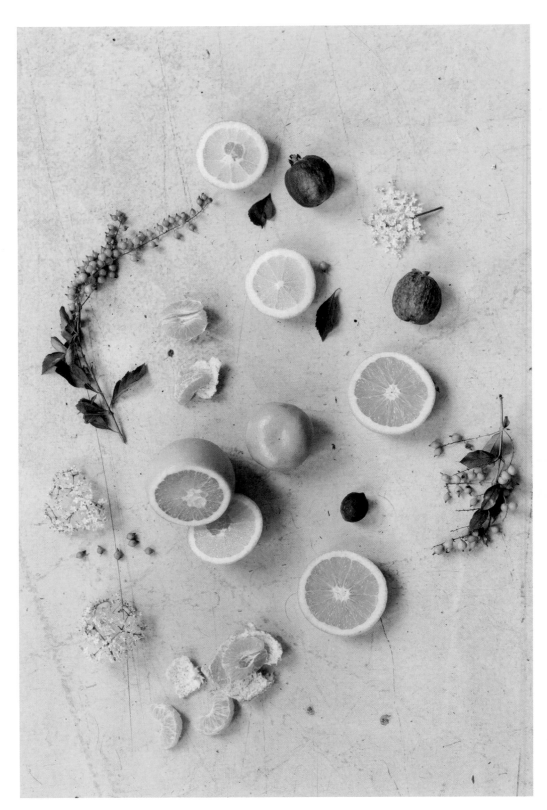

INDICATIONS YOUR LIVER MAY NEED SUPPORT

The following are symptoms that may indicate that your liver needs support:

- a liver roll (see Body Fat article on page 107)
- a tender point in the centre of your torso (which can indicate gallbladder issues, past emotional heartbreak, or massive disappointment); if your gallbladder has been removed, your liver has to make the bile on demand as the gallbladder is no longer there to store it, so additional liver support is often required
- a short fuse or bad temper, and this is new for you
- episodes or feelings of intense anger, and this is new for you
- "liverish", gritty, impatient behaviour
- premenstrual syndrome
- cellulite (can be lymphatic or cortisol-related also)
- congested skin or skin outbreaks related to the menstrual cycle
- skin rashes
- eczema, rosacea
- overheating easily
- "floaters" in your vision (these can also be a sign of iron deficiency)
- waking around 2am
- poor sleep after an evening during which you consumed alcohol
- waking up hot during the night
- not hungry for breakfast when you first get up in the morning
- a preference for coffee, not food, to start your day
- elevated cholesterol
- estrogen-dominance symptoms
- bloating easily
- daily alcohol consumption
- daily long-term caffeine consumption (although tea and green tea are more favourable than coffee, soft drinks and energy drinks).

THE TRANSFORMATION OF ESTROGEN BY THE LIVER

When a liver-loader, either consumed (exogenous) or made as a result of internal chemistry (endogenous), arrives at the front door of the liver, it has arrived to be transformed. So when any of the liver-loaders arrive at the front door of the liver, they undergo their first stage of change (phase 1 liver detoxification). Between the front door and the middle of the liver, although estrogen is still estrogen, it has been altered somewhat. This slightly changed version of estrogen then wants to go down one of the five phase 2 detox roads, and, once it has done that, it has been slightly altered again, and it is this substance that can then be excreted — expelled from your body forever.

Health problems can arise, however, when the traffic on the phase 2 pathways gets banked-up like traffic on a motorway.

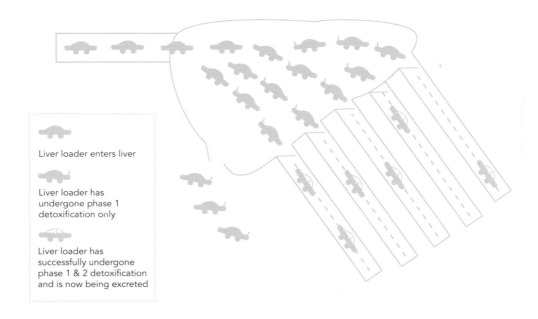

Liver loader enters liver

Liver loader has undergone phase 1 detoxification only

Liver loader has successfully undergone phase 1 & 2 detoxification and is now being excreted

After years of regularly consuming liver-loaders, and/or hormonal or bowel problems, the roads out of the liver can become congested. Conventional blood tests for liver function do not reveal this. They look at liver damage.

The liver usually takes years of battering before conventional blood tests reflect the congestion that has led to them becoming elevated (damaged) in the first place. When the traffic is banked-up, the estrogen sitting in the middle of the liver has nowhere to go, but it cannot remain waiting in the middle of the liver, as there is more rubbish constantly coming through the front door of the liver. When this occurs, the liver releases the estrogen back out into the blood, where it gets recycled. It is the recycling of these substances that can potentially be harmful to human health, including our waistlines and the risk of developing degenerative diseases due to the metabolic effects that increased levels of these substances generate. What organ can we take much better care of if we want to stop this recycling from happening? Our precious liver. Our livers need more support, and less of a load, for amazing energy, vitality and efficient fat utilization.

On another note, it is the recycled form of estrogen that is of such concern for women regarding the risk of developing reproductive cancers. Estrogen is a beautiful hormone in the right amount and with the right types of estrogen in a balanced ratio. Too much total estrogen or too much of the type linked to reproductive cancers are the problems; not only because of the estrogen itself, but also because progesterone production can never match it. That latter scenario alone can impact whether you regularly feel anxious, have a low mood, retain fluid or store body fat. Read more about this in the sex hormone sections starting on page 161.

LIVER SUPPORT

At the weekend events that I run, I help people understand the guilt that a vicious cycle of too much alcohol in the evenings, coffee to cope the next morning and sugar cravings mid-afternoon drives. The guilt you feel tends to lead you back to that cycle, whereas if you saw it as a one-off and then returned to a higher level of self-care, it would have a much more minimal impact. Remember, it is what you do every day that impacts on your health, not what you do sometimes.

Be honest with yourself about the liver-loaders in your life. Focus on taking good care of yourself and nourishing yourself, rather than on what you may need to consume less of. As you have read, the liver plays a significant role in the metabolism of countless substances that are linked to whether the body gets the message to burn body fat or store it, plus it plays a major role in disease prevention. If you eat well and move regularly but nothing ever changes with your body shape or size, or you regularly experience any of the symptoms listed above, you may find it highly beneficial to start focusing on liver support. We only have one liver. Love it accordingly.

For more ideas about how to better support your liver, explore the section about fat deposition patterns in the Body Fat article on page 107.

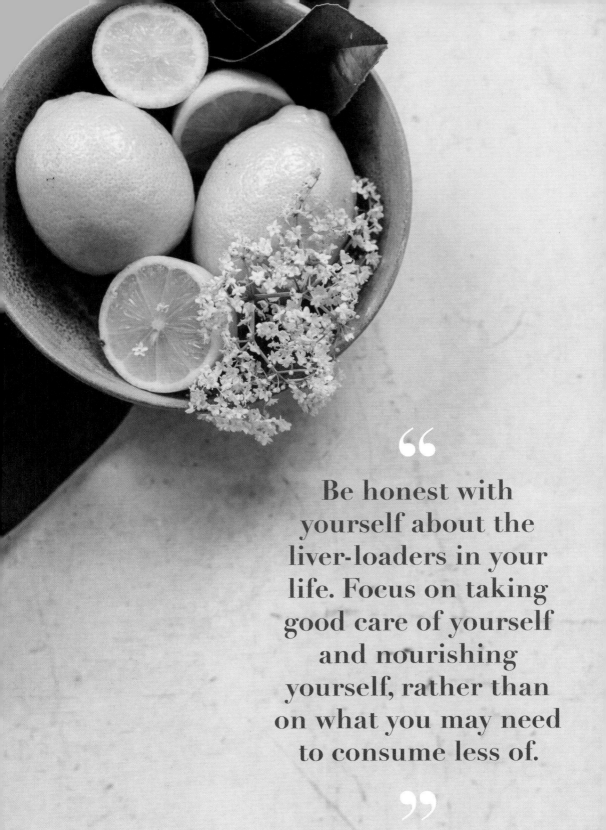

> Be honest with yourself about the liver-loaders in your life. Focus on taking good care of yourself and nourishing yourself, rather than on what you may need to consume less of.

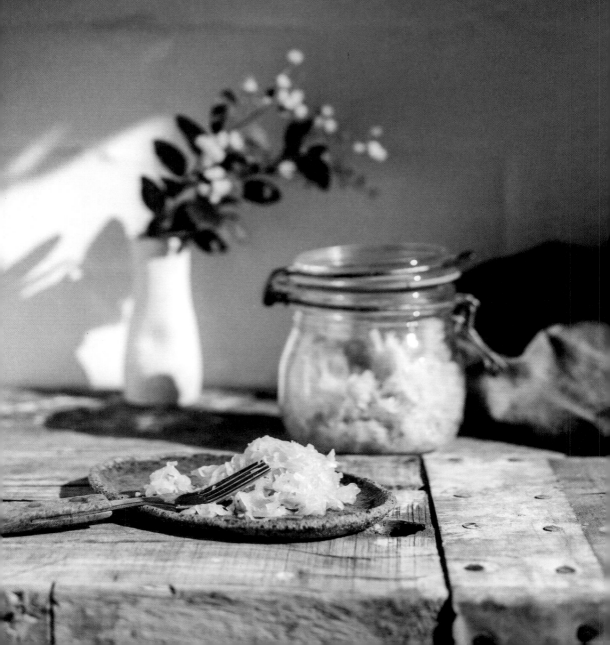

Gut bacteria

———

GUT HEALTH IS THE BASIS
OF ALL HEALTH

GUT HEALTH IS THE BASIS OF ALL HEALTH

You have about three to four kilograms of bacteria living in your large intestine, and they play a role in everything from your immune system function to your mood. They influence what calories are worth, and provide fuel to ensure that the lining of the gut remains healthy. When this balance is disturbed, health suffers and the body can present with myriad symptoms that may or may not seem directly linked to gut bacteria. Gut health is the basis of all health.

Back in the late 1990s and early 2000s, I was doing my PhD, examining the biochemical, immunological, microbiological and nutritional factors in children with autism spectrum disorder (ASD). Study participants (children with ASD, and a control group of children without ASD) supplied me with stool samples to analyse for their gut bacteria profiles. The work proved very insightful, and taught me more about the gut than I could ever have anticipated.

I saw first-hand the impact of antibiotics — no good. I saw first-hand the impact of a diet high in refined sugars and starches —

no good. I saw, too, the positive impact a change in diet could generate. Nothing else: no other intervention I was able to do came close to restoring gut health like adopting a *consistently* nutritious way of eating.

So if it means you will have better immune function, a more consistent, even, happier mood, and the ability to use body fat efficiently as a fuel, just to name a few benefits, surely you'd want to take care of it?

To do this:

- avoid antibiotics as best you can — that means only take them for your own health when you really need to, and it means eating organic meat, as sadly there are antibiotic residues in most conventional meats today

- Just Eat Real-Food — no processed foods, but plenty of vegetables and plenty of fats from a wide variety of sources; include fermented foods and bone broths, as the gut-healing components from the marrow infiltrate the soup/stew/casserole/broth.

This makes a great start to great gut health.

Cycle essentials

PUTTING THE SPOTLIGHT ON YOUR SEX HORMONES

Sex hormones have a powerful impact on how we feel, function and look, impacting on everything from whether body fat is burnt or stored, to your quality of sleep. They can impact on your mood — whether you feel anxious or calm, withdrawn or angry — and hence the food choices you make, and the way you speak to yourself and those you love the most in the world. They affect us physically and emotionally.

It is important to understand how they work in the body, as well as the healthy patterns and ratios of their production. I find that when you understand how your body works, change is more compelling and sustained. For example, rather than you feeling like someone has told you to make a change to your refined sugar intake, once you learn how your sex hormones are made and regulated by your body, and the effect on this of refined sugar, your impetus to change comes from a different place; one where sustained change is more likely. So here is how sex hormones influence your daily experience of life.

In females across their menstruation years, the ovaries are the main source of sex hormone production; however, the adrenal glands, fat cells and the liver are predominantly the other production houses of small amounts of sex hormones, too. The body also contains tissues that produce hormones themselves, but are not sensitive to hormone levels in the body. The reason some tissues are hormone-sensitive and some are not is due to the presence of receptors for a particular hormone being present on that tissue.

That means that, just because your body makes a certain hormone, doesn't mean you get the lovely or the not-so-lovely effects of the hormone. For a hormone to elicit its effects, it has to bind to a receptor. The best way to imagine the way hormones interact with a receptor site is to picture it working like a lock and a key. When they connect, you get the effects of the hormone. Breast tissue, for example, is highly sensitive to estrogen and progesterone, the two main female sex hormones, because the breasts contain receptors for both of these hormones.

Sex hormones can be delicious substances that give you energy and vitality, and yet they can also wreak havoc on your life. When it comes to a sense of calm, mental clarity, the ability to be patient and not make mountains out of molehills, fat-burning, beautiful skin, as well as fertility, very few substances in our body impact on us more than our sex hormones. The main sex hormones we will explore here are estrogen and progesterone. What occurs when they are out of balance is discussed elsewhere in the book.

ESTROGEN

Estrogen is a feminine hormone (although men naturally make it in smaller amounts), and it plays numerous important roles in the human body, including ones associated with reproduction, new bone growth, and cardiovascular health. Challenges with estrogen occur, however, when there is too much of it compared to other hormones, progesterone in particular. Estrogen can also pose a problem if there is too much of one type of estrogen compared to other types of estrogen.

The ovaries of menstruating females make estrogen, and small amounts are produced by fat cells, the adrenal glands and the liver. At menopause, ovarian production of hormones ceases.

From a reproductive perspective, estrogen's role in the female body is to lay down the lining of the uterus, and it does this between days 1 and 14 of a typical 28-day reproductive cycle, with day 1 of the cycle being the first day of menstruation. Estrogen lays the lining of the uterus down over these first 14 days to prepare the female body for a conception if it takes place. Estrogen wants a menstruating female to fall pregnant every month of her life — whether that is on her agenda or not! Remember, our bodies are completely geared for survival, and the perpetuation of the human species is a significant aspect of that survival process.

As a result of this biological imperative to conceive each month, estrogen ensures that there is adequate body fat, as most females do not immediately know when they have conceived. Without adequate body fat, it is possible that a brand-new fetus may not survive. To prevent this, estrogen signals for fat to be laid down in typically female areas, giving women a pear-like shape to better serve the childbirth process.

Estrogen is the hormone that makes female breasts bud at the first signs of puberty, broadens hips, and gives women their curves. It lays down fat on a woman's hips, bottom and thighs, and is typically responsible for making the bottom half of a female body broader than the top half. Estrogen also, unfortunately, promotes fluid retention when it is in excess, and this alone can be very stressful for a female. Her clothes don't fit her the way she would like them to, and when a woman feels "puffy and swollen" it can have a significant ripple effect on her choices for the rest of the day and night; it can affect the food choices she makes, her degree of intimacy, as well as how she speaks to herself and to those she loves the most in the world. This can add another layer of stress to what may feel like an already overwhelming life.

Sex hormones can be delicious substances that give you energy and vitality, and yet they can also wreak havoc on your life.

In a nutshell, estrogen plays many important roles in women's health. It is predominantly when there is too much of it that it poses a problem.

PROGESTERONE

Progesterone plays a variety of roles in the human body. From a reproductive perspective, its job is to hold in place the lining of the uterus that estrogen lays down between days 1 and 14 of the menstrual cycle. If the body detects that a conception has taken place, the lining of the uterus needs to be maintained and thickened, rather than shed. As a result, progesterone levels begin to rise. If there is no conception, the lining of the uterus is not needed, and progesterone levels fall away, which initiates menstruation. When health is optimal and the cycle length is 28 to 29 days, progesterone peaks seven days prior to menstruation on day 21 of cycle, and, relatively speaking, is the dominant sex hormone from just after mid-cycle until menstruation. However, this is becoming less and less common as you will see in other sections.

Biologically, progesterone has numerous other roles. It is a powerful anti-anxiety agent, an anti-depressant, a diuretic, and it is essential if you are to access fat reserves to burn for energy. Without the right amounts of progesterone across your cycle, you will predominantly utilize your glucose ("sugar"), which may lead to your body having to break down your muscle tissue for energy rather than accessing and burning fat stores; this, over time, slows your metabolic rate — not something that you want. You may also have a tendency towards an anxious or depressed mood; if you feel like you have a fortunate life and yet you still feel flat, add guilt to that emotional cocktail and a degree of confusion about what is really bothering you. You can see how layer upon layer of physical and emotional stress can form, which is a sure-fire way for women to make too many stress hormones that can also then interfere with sex hormone balance, which is explored in an upcoming section.

A menstruating female typically ovulates around day 14 of her cycle (see other sections for alternatives to this), and numerous hormonal changes occur to drive ovulation. The pituitary gland at the base of the brain sends hormonal signals to the ovary to both ripen the egg and signal its release. Follicle-stimulating hormone (FSH) stimulates the ovarian follicle, causing an egg to grow and ripen. It also triggers the production of estrogen in the follicle. This increase in estrogen tells the pituitary gland to stop producing FSH and to start making more luteinizing hormone (LH). This shift to LH causes the egg to be released from the ovary. Therefore, effective communication between the pituitary and the ovaries is essential to great reproductive health and sex hormone balance.

Estrogen wants a menstruating female to fall pregnant every month of her life — whether that is on her agenda or not!

Once the egg has been released from the ovary, a crater remains on the surface of the ovary where the egg popped out. This crater is called the corpus luteum, and this is where the bulk of a woman's progesterone is generated. As previously mentioned, progesterone is designed to peak seven days prior to the onset of menstruation — day 21 of a 28-day cycle. If conception takes place, progesterone levels need to climb to continue to hold the lining of the uterus in place. If conception does not take place during a menstrual cycle, maintaining the lining of the uterus is no longer necessary and progesterone levels fall, initiating menstruation.

It is important to note, though, that too much or too little of any hormone can pose a problem. The ratios between the amounts of different hormones can also play a role in symptom presentation. The next step is to understand whether you have too much estrogen and/or not enough progesterone, what this means, how this may have occurred, and what you can do differently in your life to balance your own sex hormones.

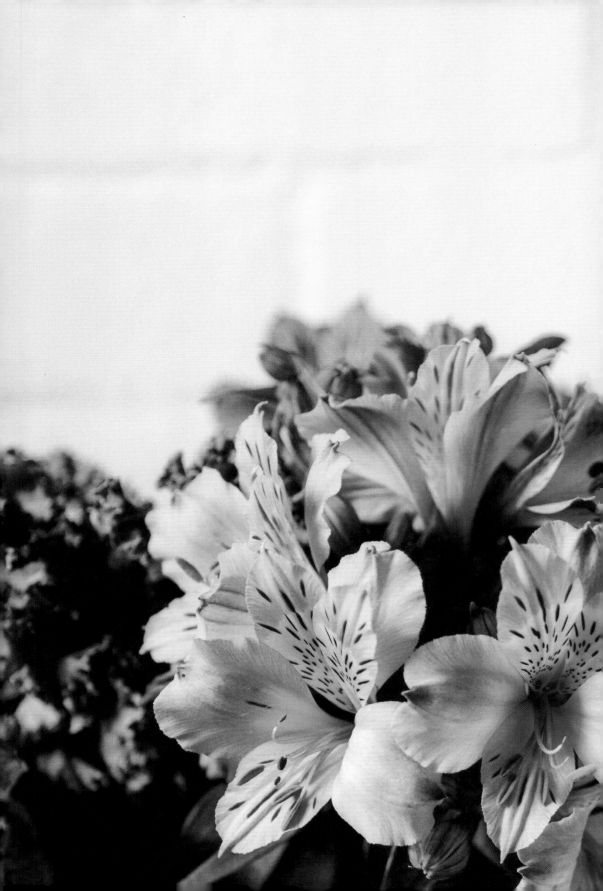

YOUR CYCLE

Across the month

DAYS 1–14
(GRAPHS 1–3)

DAYS 14–28
(GRAPHS 4–7)

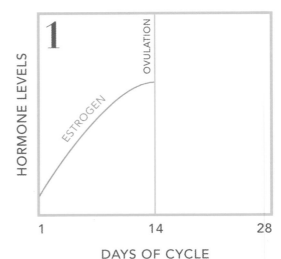

Day 1 is the first day of menstruation. Day 14 is roughly when you ovulate and day 28 is when you menstruate again. Estrogen is dominant for the first half of the cycle. It is supposed to be this way.

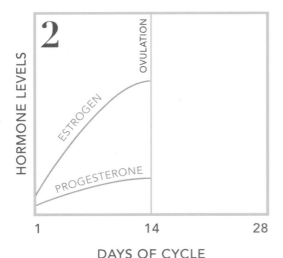

At this stage in the cycle (days 1–14), prior to ovulation, progesterone is only made by the adrenal glands.

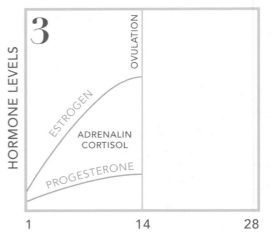

However, you also make stress hormones from the adrenals and if they are relentlessly being produced, the body gets the message that your life is in danger and that there is no food left in the world. Thinking it is doing you a favour, the body, therefore, shuts down good adrenal progesterone production. Consider the impact of this from what you are learning.

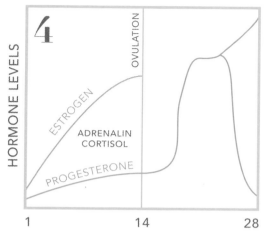

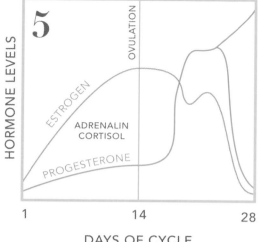

After you ovulate, you make a surge of progesterone from the corpus luteum. If there is a conception, progesterone climbs higher to maintain the endometrium. If there isn't a conception, the lining of the uterus is not needed, so progesterone falls and you menstruate.

Estrogen is secondary to (lower than) progesterone for the majority of the second half of the cycle. This picture represents healthy sex hormone balance.

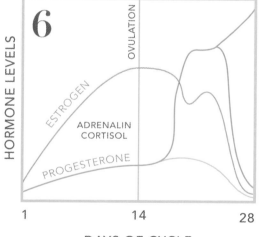

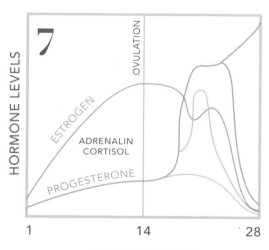

If you don't ovulate, you rely entirely on the adrenal production of progesterone. Yet, if you are stressed, the line representing progesterone could be flat lined across the bottom of the graph.

Or you may ovulate, but you don't make optimal amounts of progesterone so it is only dominant over estrogen for a few days of the second half of the cycle. This means estrogen is dominant leading into the menstrual period. This is one of the most common sex hormone pictures that causes the symptoms of PMT.

Hormone disruption

THE INTERACTION BETWEEN SEX HORMONES AND STRESS HORMONES

The relationship between sex hormones and stress hormones is a fascinating and powerful one, and it is critical for people to understand it for their health and happiness now, as well as in the future.

As you now understand, estrogen is the dominant sex hormone between day 1 and day 14 of the menstrual cycle. For the first half of the menstrual cycle, a relatively small amount of progesterone is made from the adrenal glands. For the sake of this description, let's call the amount two units. Remember, the reproductive role of progesterone is to hold in place the lining of the uterus, with the additional biological functions of it being an anti-anxiety agent, an anti-depressant and a diuretic.

However, your adrenal glands are also where you make your stress hormones, namely adrenalin and cortisol. The body makes adrenalin after the consumption of caffeine or as a result of the perception of pressure and urgency. Adrenalin communicates to every cell of your body that your life is in danger, even though all you may have done is had an intense conversation with a colleague and/or mindlessly consumed three coffees this morning. My point is to highlight that both physical (for example, caffeine consumption) and emotional (for example, a perception of pressure or a misunderstanding from an argument) processes can drive adrenalin production and communicate that danger is present.

Cortisol is the long-term, chronic stress hormone. When you are internally rattled, cortisol communicates to every cell in your body that there is no food left in the world, and as a result it wants your body to break down muscle and store fat to get you through the lean times it perceives lie ahead. Even though food is abundant for you, and your cortisol production is likely to be coming from areas of your life about which you feel uncertain (such as your finances or relationships), your body relates it to the historical causes of long-term stress and an ensuing threat to the food supply.

Adrenalin communicates to every cell of your body that your life is in danger.

Since your body links progesterone to fertility, if your body perceives that your life is under threat and that there is no food left in the world, the last thing it wants is for you to bring a baby into that world, so it shuts down the adrenal production of progesterone, thinking it is doing you a great, big favour. Estrogen and cortisol, both signalling fat storage and ongoing stress, remain, while you have lost the counterbalancing hormone that helps keep you calm and not anxious, and helps burn fat and get rid of excess fluid.

In my opinion, the shift away from good adrenal progesterone production, due to the constant production of stress hormones, and the metabolic and biological consequences of this, is one of the biggest challenges facing Western women's health today. I spoke about it in my TEDx talk, and this whole scenario tends to create a major "a-ha!" moment for women attending my weekend events.

This situation alone is a modern-day, monumental shift in female chemistry, and it can torment a woman's emotional and physical wellbeing. This shift plays an enormous role in whether you feel vital and alive, or whether you have to drag yourself through each day, and why you might feel a need to do everything with urgency. A female can go from feeling happy, healthy, balanced and energized, with great clarity of mind and an even mood,

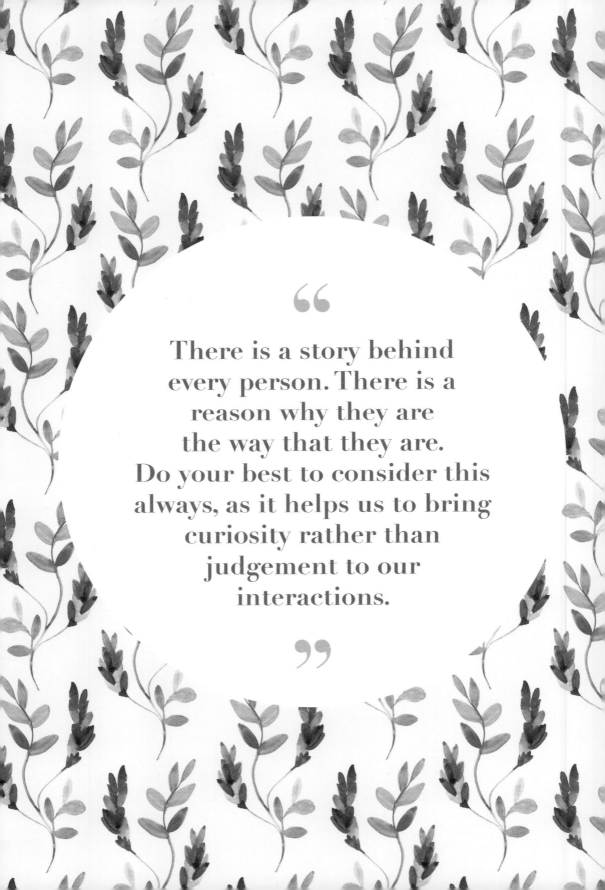

> " "
>
> There is a story behind every person. There is a reason why they are the way that they are. Do your best to consider this always, as it helps us to bring curiosity rather than judgement to our interactions.
>
> " "

to having a foggy brain and feeling either overly anxious about things she cannot name, or utterly exhausted, as a result of this shift to constant stress hormone production and the subsequent low level (or absence) of progesterone. Physically, at times, she may feel puffy, heavy, bloated and full of fluid, with a sense that her clothes are getting tighter by the minute no matter what she eats, whether this is actually true or not.

Poor adrenal production of progesterone needs to be addressed.

Here are some things to consider embracing in your life to help that happen:

- Breathe diaphragmatically: as you slowly inhale through your nostrils, your tummy sticks out; no need to hold your breath, simply pause, and then slowly exhale as your tummy moves back in toward your spine. Nothing lowers stress hormones faster than diaphragmatically breathing. Breathing this way most of the time communicates safety to your body, lowering stress hormone levels and allowing the body to feel safe enough to produce progesterone again. This may mean attending regular classes of a breath-focused practice such as t'ai chi, qi gong, pilates, yoga, restorative yoga or Stillness Through Movement and/or simply creating moments throughout the day when you check in to notice how you are breathing. For example, while you wait for the kettle to boil in the morning, when you are stopped at traffic lights, or every hour on the hour at your desk. Create rituals in your day that help you to become breath-aware and allow this to permeate each and every day. Save the short, sharp, shallow breaths (driven by adrenalin) for only when you really need them.

- Herbs such as licorice help the adrenals to be more adaptive to stress and help restore their function if they are depleted, while paeonia helps foster efficient communication between the pituitary and the ovaries and helps to balance the ratio of FSH to LH, again fostering regular ovulation, and hence enhanced progesterone production.

A NEW BABY

Another scenario where stress hormones can abound and interfere with sex hormones is after the delivery of a baby. Once the placenta has formed by week 12 of gestation, progesterone levels climb to around 300 to 400 units. Pregnancy is the time when a woman has the highest level of circulating progesterone, which is why many women glow, especially from the second trimester onwards. Once a woman has birthed the placenta, however, her progesterone level plunges from 400 to zero! Fortunately, birth brings on some other feel-good hormones, such as oxytocin, although they tend to be more short-lived.

Historically, babies were welcomed into extended families and communities. Today, a more common scenario (but not the only scenario) is a hospital birth followed by a new mother being at home alone with her newborn during the day while her partner continues to work to pay the mortgage and other bills. If there are challenges in their relationship, or challenges caused by the needs of other children, financial stress, ill or aging parents, an unwell newborn or simply one who won't sleep, the new home environment with baby can be highly stressful. Another common stressful scenario is where a new mother has made what she thought would be a welcome transition (temporarily or permanently) from a corporate career to staying at home with her baby, but is now second-guessing her decision. The guilt and confusion around this scenario can be overwhelming. Such scenarios do not promote the restoration of adrenal progesterone levels, as the body is so busy making stress hormones

Pregnancy is the time when a woman has the highest level of circulating progesterone, which is why many women glow, especially from the second trimester onwards.

that it is not "safe" for the new mum to make the fertility-linked progesterone.

Remember, progesterone is one of the most powerful anti-anxiety and anti-depressant substances the body makes. On the other hand, if mum and baby do have support, and the new mum doesn't feel she is alone with her new precious bundle — whether this is simply due to the mother's beliefs, attitudes and perceptions, or her actual physical support from other people — then adrenal progesterone levels are far more likely to be restored, and her chemistry is all the better for it.

If you are reading this, you have a child/children and you are struggling, please seek support; physical (such as good-quality nutritional and/or herbal medicine, and doing yoga, for example) and/or emotional.

You may also like to read about post-natal depletion in my book *Exhausted to Energized.*

The highs and lows

TOO MUCH ESTROGEN? NOT ENOUGH PROGESTERONE? OR BOTH?

There are many poor-health scenarios that have become all too common. This does not, however, make them normal. Challenges with the menstrual cycle fall into this category. Your periods are supposed to just turn up. No pain, no cramps, no clots, no tender breasts, no mood swings. Anything else is just feedback… Feedback asking you to make some different choices about how you eat, drink, move, think, breathe, believe and/or perceive. And it's feedback you want to act on.

There are a number of scenarios that can create these symptoms, with the most common ones involving too much estrogen and not enough progesterone, or, for more and more women, both. In both of these situations estrogen is in excess — or estrogen dominance as it is often referred to — but there's more you need to know in order to decipher what might be going on for you.

THE CYCLE

Estrogen is supposed to be the dominant sex hormone for the first half of the cycle. This is known as the follicular phase. Small amounts of progesterone will be made by the adrenals glands at this stage, but not yet from the ovaries. Progesterone is only made from the ovaries after ovulation, in what is known as the luteal phase. The crater that remains on the surface of the ovary after ovulation — the corpus luteum — is the main producer of progesterone across the menstruation years, and it is designed to be dominant for the majority of the second half of the cycle. To be precise, you make progesterone from the ovary from which you ovulate (and only if you ovulate) for the final 10 to 14 days of your cycle. This means that on day 21 of the cycle your progesterone will peak if you have a 28-day cycle. If your cycle is longer, and it tends to be more like 36 days, you may not start producing progesterone until day 22. My goal for people is to help their body menstruate every 28–29 days, without discomfort; I have witnessed women with cycles 35 days, or longer, establish and maintain a 28–29-day cycle through nutrition and lifestyle changes. The body is truly breathtaking.

Knowing where you are at in your cycle is essential to great health and to resolving any challenges with sex hormone production and/or balance. Keeping track of when you menstruate and any symptoms you may experience at this time really helps you, and a health professional you may work with, to be precise about where to focus to get the outcomes you are seeking, such as resolving premenstrual tension (PMT).

The best day to test progesterone is seven days before your period. Keep in mind, if you have blood or saliva tests for sex hormones, that you will need to know what day in your cycle you are at, because if progesterone is tested before you ovulate (in the follicular phase) then it will be very low, as it is supposed to be at this stage. However, if you have your progesterone tested and you are in your luteal phase, if you know you have ovulated a minimum of three days prior to the test, or if you noted that your period arrived within 10 days of doing the test, then it needs to be nice and high. Just so you know, your temperature will also tend to increase after you have ovulated.

One of the topics I cover in detail at my *Beautiful You Weekends* is sex hormone balance. And one of the stand-out conversations for all groups over the years is this one: you need to know if you have low progesterone or no progesterone, and here's why: you need to know whether you are ovulating or not. Conventional medicine teaches that if you did ovulate, your blood (serum) progesterone will be at 20–25 nmol/L (units), and it teaches that if it is lower than that, it means you haven't ovulated — known as an anovular cycle — or the timing of the test was incorrect to effectively measure progesterone (ie, not done seven days prior to when menstruation would typically occur). However, I have not seen this to be the case in clinical practice. On day 21 of a 28-day cycle, I have had six women with 25 units of progesterone. Some have had 10 units, which to me indicates that they are ovulating, but they are poor progesterone-producers at that time. Therefore, they have low progesterone. Clinically, if a woman has a luteal-phase progesterone level between 10 and 25, she has ovulated, but the lower that number, the more major her symptoms will be.

NO OVULATION MEANS NO PROGESTERONE

However, if the luteal-phase (day 21 of a 28-day cycle) level of progesterone is less than 10 units, this suggests that the woman has not ovulated. And this must be addressed. It is critical for you to know (and often the assistance of a health professional is required) why you are not ovulating, rather than just be treated for "low progesterone". Simply treating low progesterone in this case won't resolve what is really going on: anovulatory cycles. Helping the body to re-establish an ovulation pattern will, amongst other benefits, generate a healthier progesterone level.

In my experience, no ovulation occurs when:
- there is a consistent, relentless output of stress hormones
- polycystic ovarian syndrome (PCOS) is present, or
- there is poor thyroid function (this is not necessary a thyroid disease, but the thyroid gland is not working optimally).

The reason why you aren't ovulating needs to be determined, as that is what needs addressing.

LOW PROGESTERONE

If you are ovulating and your luteal-phase progesterone level is only just 10 units but not much more than that, then you will typically feel highly anxious, have a low mood, and feel like you can't get your breath past your heart in the lead-up to menstruation. You may also have premenstrual spotting, heavy bleeding and PMT. If you have low progesterone, then you will need to increase it to feel better. To do that, the focus needs to be on supporting the health of the ovarian follicles themselves. Getting optimal amounts of the nutrients that the ovaries need to correct functioning is essential.

These include:

- iodine
- selenium
- zinc, and
- magnesium.

It is very important to address inflammation, which may involve dietary changes. There are some beautiful medicinal herbs, such as licorice and paeonia, that work in a multitude of ways to support a healthy cycle. The herbal medicine chaste tree, also known as vitex, can be helpful for some women, while it doesn't suit others. A medical herbalist can guide you with this.

When I work with people, I pay attention to what their bodies are communicating via symptoms as the first port of call. Tests can be highly insightful, of course, but it is what the body is demonstrating that I focus on. As progesterone levels can fluctuate over a two-hour period, symptoms matter first, and tests are not always needed, particularly if you work with an experienced health professional.

ESTROGEN

Too much estrogen is not good for health. Estrogen in the right amounts and the right types is highly beneficial, as it is great for bones and heart health, and has been shown to improve insulin sensitivity. In the first half of the cycle, the main form of estrogen — estradiol — will be slowly rising towards its peak, which occurs a few days prior to ovulation. After ovulation it slowly starts to decrease again, while progesterone levels are supposed to increase.

However, when estrogen levels are too high at any stage of the cycle, it is usually the result of the liver recycling estrogen, rather than detoxifying it. The liver has to change estrogen before it can be eliminated, but if the biochemical pathways for estrogen detoxification are congested and are too busy dealing with other "liver-loaders", then the estrogen gets recycled. A major problem, however, is that the form that gets recycled is the one typically linked to reproductive cancers. When a woman has the symptoms of too much estrogen — which are typically heavy, clotty, painful periods, swollen, tender, congested breasts, and mood swings that usually involve irritability and/or sadness — it is liver health that must be addressed. In this case, you are estrogen-dominant, due to the liver not keeping up with the estrogen being generated inside you from the ovaries, adrenals and body fat cells, as well as from the environment's plastics and pesticides. You may also have less progesterone than is ideal for you, and this, too, makes you estrogen-dominant, but in this case it is due to not ovulating or the ovary being a poor progesterone producer. While they are separate scenarios (excess estrogen and low/no progesterone), they can occur at the same time. If that is the case, the liver, the adrenals and the ovarian follicles need to be supported.

How do you support healthy estrogen detoxification via the liver? Here are some simple ways for you to consider incorporating into your lifestyle:

- incorporate the Brassica genus of vegetables in your diet. These include broccoli, cauliflower, kale, cabbage, Brussels sprouts. Broccoli sprouts contain some of the highest levels of the substances you need for efficient estrogen detoxification, and are a great daily inclusion in your meals and/or nutritional supplements

- you might like to try our Brilliant Brassica Soup, available from the recipe section at *www.drlibby.com*

- using turmeric is another way to support the liver

detoxification pathways. Use it in cooking and/or include it in your nutritional supplements

- dandelion is a wonderful liver support. Enjoy a daily tea ritual, or include it in your nutritional supplements

- increase the plant food content of what you eat on a daily basis, as the liver utilizes substances unique to plants for detoxification, beyond just the vitamins and minerals they contain

- increase the antioxidant content of what you eat on a daily basis, because, during the liver's detoxification processes, what are known as reactive oxygen species (ROS) are thrown off. You need additional antioxidants to mop them up so that they don't damage your tissues, which is one of the ways we age from the inside out. Antioxidants are found predominantly in coloured plant foods. Berries and blackcurrants are particularly high in some superstar antioxidants

- be honest with yourself about how many liver-loaders you are consuming. Do you need to consume less alcohol, for example? Or take a break from it for two menstrual cycles? Be honest with yourself about your first response to this question

- include good-quality herbal medicine such as St Mary's thistle and globe artichoke on a daily basis to support healthy bile production, which is essential for effective detoxification and the elimination of estrogen.

Cramps and confusion

REPRODUCTIVE SYSTEM CHALLENGES

The menstrual cycle is a stunning barometer for what is going on inside the body. However, the wake-up calls can be relatively gentle or can scream loudly at you. Let's explore some of the most common reproductive system challenges, what might be occurring, and the options to change this.

PMT, PERIOD PAIN AND CRAMPING

What might be causing these symptoms?
- too much estrogen
    - usually requires liver support
- not enough progesterone
    - usually requires adrenal/stress support and/or ovarian follicle support
- no progesterone
    - usually due to anovulatory cycles, so adrenal/stress and or thyroid and/or pituitary to ovarian communication needs support
- inflammation
    - usually due to a poor-quality diet, too high in processed foods, and poor gut health and/or stress
- magnesium deficiency.

HOW DO I SUPPORT MY BODY WITH THIS?

Dietary changes that may be required are highly individual. They usually involve exploring how foods and drinks containing gluten, casein, caffeine, alcohol, sugar and other processed foods affect you. Good-quality herbal medicine is often highly effective at supporting the restoration of biochemical pathways so that symptoms resolve.

Here are some examples:

- too much estrogen
  - liver support, such as herbal medicine containing broccoli sprouts, turmeric and dandelion
- not enough progesterone
  - ovarian and adrenal support, such as herbal medicine containing licorice, paeonia, iodine and selenium
- no progesterone
  - why you aren't ovulating needs to be determined (see other sections in the book for more information).

ENDOMETRIOSIS AND PRE-MENSTRUAL MIGRAINE

Both of these conditions are linked to an excess of estrogen. For the majority of clients I have worked with who were experiencing them, the following combination has resolved the pain in most cases.

Dairy-free (casein-free) eating; gluten-free is sometimes warranted as a trial as well if there is an existing autoimmune condition, or a strong Irish heritage (explained in a separate section)

- no coffee
- no alcohol
- no sugar
- herbs for liver support, containing broccoli sprouts, turmeric and dandelion
- anti-inflammatory fats such as those found in flaxseeds, chia seeds, walnuts, pecans and oily fish.

Stress management is often also necessary, such as a 10-minute restorative yoga practice each evening before bed. This may simply be "legs up the wall" for 10 minutes while you diaphragmatically breathe.

POLYCYSTIC OVARIAN SYNDROME (PCOS)

In PCOS, the signals from the pituitary to the ovaries asking an egg to ripen and then be released aren't effective, so ova (eggs) ripen on the surface of the ovary and form cysts. The focus needs to be on re-establishing good pituitary–ovarian communication to foster regular ovulation. Where the person perceives there is stress in their life must be explored. As well as exploring their beliefs and their stress, individualised dietary changes are often needed to help mitigate insulin resistance and inflammation.

Herbs that are beneficial are those that support the adrenals (stress) and pituitary–ovarian communication, which include licorice, paeonia and chaste tree. Thyroid function also needs to be investigated. Nutrients that support healthy thyroid function include iodine, selenium and iron.

Just because it isn't happening right now, doesn't mean it never will.

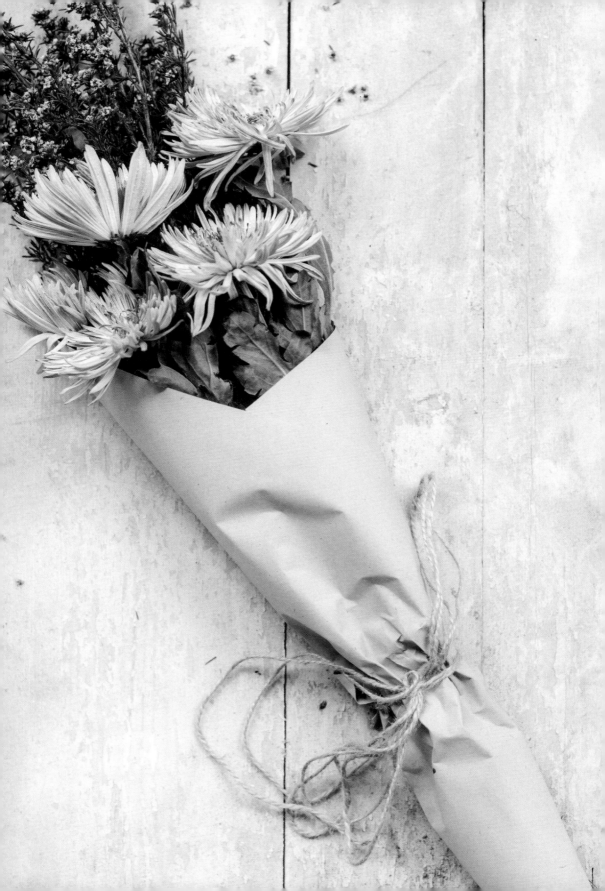

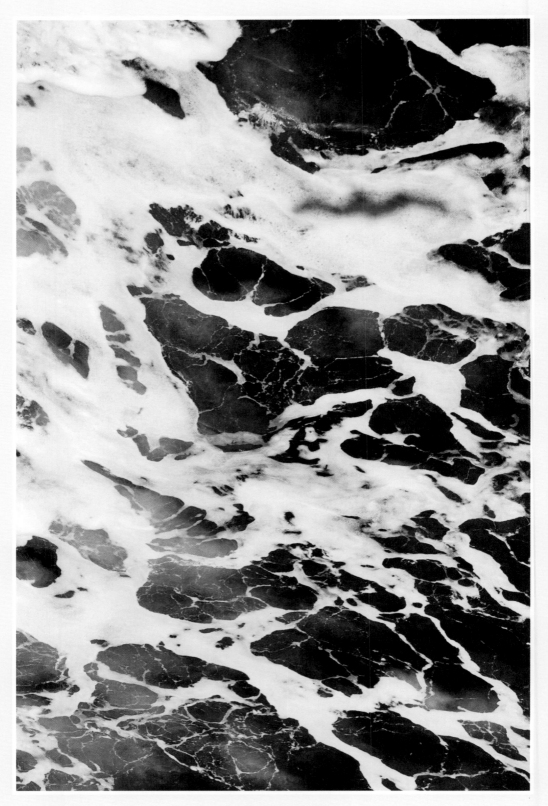

Women's Wellness Wisdom

Fluid retention
HOW TO MINIMIZE IT

Many women feel that they are fat when really they are either bloated or retaining fluid. I never weigh clients, and I don't encourage them to weigh themselves. I do this for many reasons, but one is that as hormone levels fluctuate over the month (and even over a day), so can the amounts of fluid being retained, until the hormones return to balance. Besides, when you weigh yourself, remember that all you are really weighing is your self-esteem. I have met thousands of women who can gain three kilograms in a day — and to say that this messes with their minds is an understatement. If you get on the scales in the morning and weigh 70 kilograms, and by the evening you weigh 73 kilograms, especially if you have eaten well and exercised that day (and even if you haven't eaten well or exercised that day), it is easy to feel incredibly disheartened and wonder how on Earth this could possibly happen. Weight can feel like just another thing to worry and panic about, which does little to help with your weight loss, given the stress hormones this will likely lead you to generate!

Remember this: it is not physically possible to gain three kilograms of body fat in a single day. The only possible cause is fluid retention. Yet, even though the logical part of the mind knows this, seeing three extra kilos on the scales over the course of just a day, or even a week, will make most women, no matter how reasonable they are, feel anxious, impatient, frustrated and generally lousy. And are they more likely to make good or poor food choices when they feel this way? All of this always feels worse if they have been eating well and exercising and are still gaining weight, as then they tend to think that this must mean that they have to find the time to do even more exercise, but they don't know where on Earth that time is going to come from because they are already stretched for time.

There can be numerous factors behind fluid retention, and if it is significant and goes on for too long it is best to see your GP.

Essentially, fluid retention can be driven by:

- poor lymphatic flow
- a congested liver from too many liver-loaders
- excess estrogen, usually due to poor liver detoxification
- mineral deficiencies and imbalances
- poor thyroid function, or
- poor progesterone production.

From an energy medicine perspective, I also encourage you to think about who or what you may be holding on to that no longer serves you. Perhaps it is a belief or perception that no longer supports you, and your body is simply trying to wake you up to this and get you to change. So many of us fear change, whether we realize this or not.

Excess estrogen can be another likely culprit when it comes to fluid retention. It can also drive headaches, including migraines, increase blood clotting, decrease libido, interfere with thyroid hormone production, and, due to its relationship with progesterone, lead us to feel like we have to do everything with haste. These are big health consequences, all because there is too much of one little hormone.

If you retain fluid, there is no one-size-fits-all solution.

You need to apply the solutions based on the cause, on the mechanism that is creating the fluid retention.

For poor lymphatic flow, try:

- rebounding on a mini-trampoline
- exercise (but don't run long distances)
- diaphragmatic breathing
- lymphatic massage
- St Mary's thistle (a herbal medicine)

For a congested liver from too many liver-loaders, try:

- consuming less alcohol, caffeine, refined and artificial sugars, trans fats, processed foods, preservatives – or take a break from all of them and Just Eat Real Food
- swapping what you clean your house with for proven ecologically sound products
- swapping what you put on your skin for proven ecologically sound products
- limiting consumption of pesticides by choosing organic foods
- limiting the use of non-essential medications, such as for headache relief – do your best to get to the heart of why you get headaches if you get them regularly, for example
- incorporating St Mary's thistle, globe artichoke and turmeric in your diet, as they are brilliant and effective herbs for supporting liver detoxification pathways
- amping up the vegetable content of your diet, particularly the Brassica genus of vegetables; Broccoli sprouts , in particular, are highly effective at enhancing liver detoxification pathways

Where there is excess estrogen, apply the liver support strategies, as the excess is usually due to the poor liver detoxification of estrogen, and the estrogen is being recycled. Where there is poor progesterone production, refer to the section that helps you discern between low and no progesterone production. Where there is poor thyroid function, refer to the thyroid information.

For mineral deficiencies and imbalances, try:

- increasing your magnesium intake, which is found in green leafy vegetables, nuts and seeds, and/or take a good-quality supplement
- significantly reducing or eliminating processed food in your diet, as it contains an excess of poor-quality salt
- swapping any salt you add at home to a good-quality salt that contains a broad range of minerals in trace amounts, such as Celtic sea salt or Himalayan salt — and be sure that any salt you use contains iodine (this will be written on the label).

Menopause

Menopause is a natural process within a women's life, yet it can be a strikingly different experience for each person. The symptoms of menopause are as varied and as individual as the menstrual cycle itself. Some women transition from regular menstrual flow to the cessation of their periods and beyond with little or no challenging symptoms, while for others it is a time of insomnia, hot flushes, constant heat, low mood, no libido and/or weight gain. Any or all of these experiences may lead to strained relationships in both family and career, yet this doesn't have to be the case. Challenging symptoms of menopause are just another way the body is asking you to make some changes to your choices, and instead the transition into the post-menopausal years can be one of renewed vigour and personal growth.

Fundamentally, menopause (the cessation of the menstrual cycle) means that the ovaries cease their production of sex hormones — predominantly estrogen and progesterone. Small amounts are still made in other areas of the body, by the adrenal glands, liver and body fat cells, for example. Physically and emotionally, however, this transition can be life-changing in more ways than simply not menstruating anymore. Symptoms primarily arise from hormonal decline, but factors such as physiology (particularly muscle mass), organ function (particularly the liver and adrenals), lifestyle, diet and health history, and emotions can play a role, too.

The relentless output of stress hormones in the lead-up to menopause — or, for too many women these days, this has gone on for decades — can lead to some of the most debilitating symptoms. If your adrenals glands have been receiving the message that they need to churn out stress

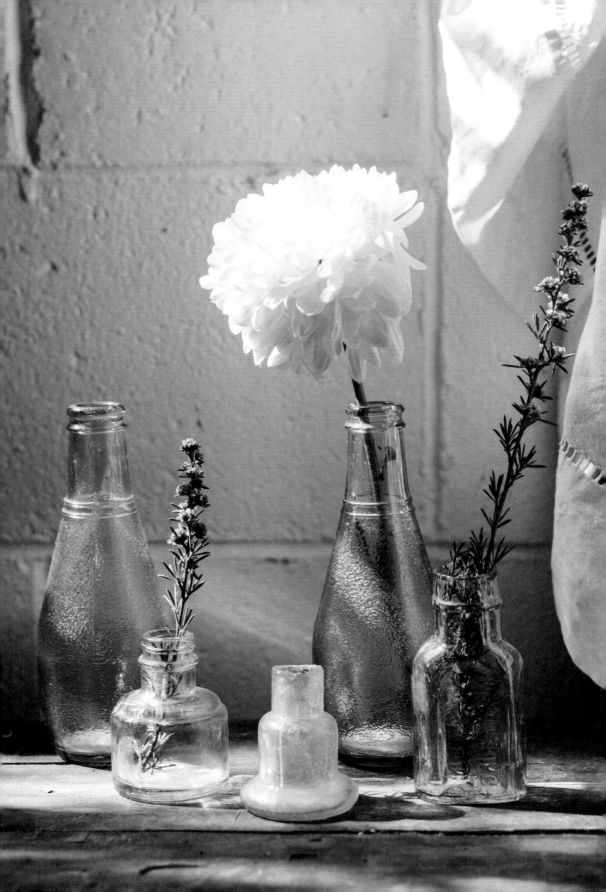

hormones, due to genuine stress, excess caffeine consumption, or from the perception of pressure and urgency, then they won't have efficiently made sex hormones across that time. When menopause hits (that is, when no more ovarian hormones are produced), you are supposed to predominantly rely on adrenal hormones — yet you may not have made sex hormones from your adrenals for a very long time. So instead of going from having bucket-loads of hormones to a small amount, you virtually go from having plenty to none. Couple this with a liver that has likely been in overdrive trying to deal with the liver-loaders many people ingest or absorb these days, and you have a cocktail for sleeplessness and debilitating body heat.

The transition to post-menopause can take several years, and this is referred to as perimenopause, when hormonal output gradually reduces over time. This can initially cause irregularity in the period frequency and flow, and associated premenstrual symptoms. For some, blood flow becomes increasingly heavier, whereas for others the flow is reduced and they experience fewer symptoms. Once the ovaries cease the production of hormones entirely, small amounts of estrogen and progesterone are supposed to be made by the adrenal glands, which act to protect against a degenerative disease associated with bone density and cardiovascular decline; yet to reiterate, for many women the consistent and relentless output of stress hormones means that this hasn't happened for many years leading into menopause.

The health and function of the adrenal glands play a major role in determining how the transition of menopause affects us.

The health and function of the adrenal glands, therefore, play a major role in determining how the transition of menopause affects us. Another thing to consider is, if the adrenals aren't up to the task of overseeing the production of yet another hormone, what happens then? The body always has a Plan B, and in menopause the body fat acts as a production facility for estrogen while the ovaries shut up shop and the adrenals try to take over. If the adrenals don't have the resources to help, body fat may increase in an attempt to help out... Here's yet another example of how the calorie concept as the sole determinant of body size is a myth.

The number one priority here is to manage stress. Creating calm in our life, despite what external circumstances ask of us, is an essential life skill these days. Whatever this may mean for you, do it. Meditation and yoga are two powerful breath-focused practices that can support the body to transition from a dominant sympathetic nervous system (fight or flight) to the calm parasympathetic nervous system (rest and repair). Diaphragmatic breathing (moving your tummy in and out as you breathe) reduces stress hormone output significantly, and takes the pressure off the adrenal glands.

A balanced and functional approach to movement is critical — combining restorative movement such as yoga, pilates and qi gong with resistance training and gentle weight strengthening is particularly important for the metabolic rate. Metabolism through menopause may decrease by 10 to 15 per cent; this is more significant if muscle mass going into menopause is low. It is important to take that into consideration and keep metabolism sustained through building muscle, eating regularly, and focusing on whole, unprocessed foods devoid of refined sugars and trans fatty acids. Healthy fats are vital, as well: to synthesize hormones, we need varied essential fats, such as oily fish, flaxseeds, chia seeds, walnuts, pecans, evening primrose oil, blackcurrant oil or borage oil. Avocados and macadamia nuts (and their oils) are also a great choice. They are also very satiating and can help to regulate blood glucose levels.

Essential fatty acids from the aforementioned healthy fats are a critical part of keeping our hair, skin and nails healthy, too. They are of particular importance if you are experiencing hair thinning and brittle or dry nails. Nutrients such as magnesium, calcium and vitamin D are often used to help manage hot flushes, and sleep and mood disturbance; however, most importantly they can help to preserve bone density. Zinc is also hugely important to help synthesize sex hormones and regulate cholesterol metabolism, which can often increase as hormonal production declines and the liver has more to deal with.

Holistically, each person tends to require an individualized plan, detailing food, movement, stress management, specific nutrients if required, and potentially herbal medicine — particularly when there are hot flushes and/or sleep issues. Medicinal herbs have a unique advantage in that they modulate rather than stimulate a physical response. This means that they adjust to the body's forever-changing environment by acting on hormone receptors to trigger a particular response.

Remember that hormonal production varies daily, if not hourly, according to what is required to sustain a balanced system, to sustain homeostasis. This is particularly relevant in perimenopause when the ovaries are still producing hormones, albeit in much lower quantities than previously, and thus the internal environment is in constant state of flux. Post-menopausally, the hormonal output is not as varied and thus requires a different approach.

When formulating a herbal tonic for someone, there is always much to take into consideration, and this needs to be assessed on an individual basis, to make it as effective as possible. Herbs work well synergistically with other herbs, and they can affect different body systems simultaneously. Wild yam, for example, reduces inflammation, reduces spasms and cramping, and modulates estrogen by acting on specific

Creating calm in our life, despite what external circumstances ask of us, is an essential life skill these days.

estrogen receptors. Each herb can help stabilize a different symptom. Please note, this is for educational purposes; this is not prescriptive. Herbal medicine must be tailored to individual needs by a qualified health professional. An example of a formula for someone with hot flushes, difficulty sleeping, low mood, low energy and cravings for alcohol may look something like this:

- plants in the Schisandra genus
    - to provide liver support and cooling for hormonal hot flushes
- rhodiola
    - to help with mood, cravings and energy levels, it is an excellent adrenal herb
- wild yam
    - to modulate the estrogen and help relax the body
- St John's wort
    - can be helpful for mood regulation due to the reduction in serotonin (our happy, calm and content hormone) that can occur with reduced estrogen output.

Other helpful herbs include rehmannia, black cohosh, withania and/or milk thistle. Always seek advice from a qualified practitioner who can make a specific formula to suit your needs and understand where in the menopause journey you may be.

Lastly, but certainly not least, supporting optimal liver function is vital in the transition to menopause to help manage hot flushes and sleep. Broccoli sprouts and turmeric can be highly beneficial across this time. Be mindful of liver-loaders, such as coffee and alcohol, and take care to avoid synthetic chemicals that may be present in cleaning products, cosmetics and processed foods.

There is a growing body of evidence to suggest that we are being exposed to many endocrine-disrupting substances in our current environment, so whenever and wherever possible make a concerted effort to choose natural and organic options. When it comes to this transition, don't be afraid to seek help: your journey doesn't have to be one of suffering. In fact, make it a time in your life when you thrive. Use the feedback from your body to make the changes it requires from you in your lifestyle choices.

Remember, challenging symptoms of menopause are just another way the body is asking you to make some changes to your choices. If you are currently experiencing uncomfortable perimenopause or menopause symptoms, then use the guide below to help you understand the areas you may need to focus on:

SYMPTOMS	AREAS TO FOCUS ON
Insomnia	Liver Nervous system Adrenals
Hot flushes	Gut Liver Adrenals
Constant heat	Gut Liver
Low mood	Gut Adrenals Thyroid
No libido	Nervous system Adrenals
Weight gain	Gut Liver Nervous system Adrenals Thyroid

If you are perimenopausal or post-menopausal, is it smooth sailing for you? If so, wonderful! If not, where do you feel you need to focus? Capture new choices you can make that can better support you at this time.

Movement

CREATING STRENGTH, FLEXIBILITY AND RESTORATION

Do you think even 100 years ago people woke up and thought "Great! Off for a 20-kilometre run today!" Not likely. I believe that for people in the West, when the calorie equation was presented as being the only mechanism through which we burn or store fat (a myth), the concept of running long distances to burn calories was born. In other words, it was born from a world of excess.

Of course we are designed to move, and research and common sense teach us that a sedentary lifestyle takes years off our lives, not to mention negatively affecting the quality of our lives. We need to move. However, when you run long distances, you generate a huge amount of free radicals. This means you need huge numbers of antioxidants to mop these up so that your tissues aren't damaged, and so that aging and degeneration processes aren't over-stimulated. The wear and tear on your joints and ligaments can also be challenging to motion in the long term. Plus, you need to embrace muscle-building exercise as well, because running long distances is catabolic, meaning you break muscles down. This does not support your metabolic rate in the long term. Now, I am not saying don't run if you love it. If you feel energized and uplifted at the end of it, that's wonderful. I am simply pointing out that it is not the ultimate exercise that too many people still think it is today. In fact, unless you are taking other lifestyle steps to combat the effects of the long-distance running, you may be doing more harm than good. Try interval training instead – short bursts of running, if you enjoy it.

Without a functional body, you can miss the joy, freedom and independence of simple pleasures.

Also consider that unless we actively build muscle from the age of 30 onwards, we lose it. Embrace resistance training. This doesn't have to mean going to gym unless that spins your tyres. In a yoga practice, you resist your own body weight. Pilates, too, is excellent resistance training, as is walking, gardening, farm work, carrying groceries and children. Don't avoid movement. Take the stairs regularly, for example. Build muscle.

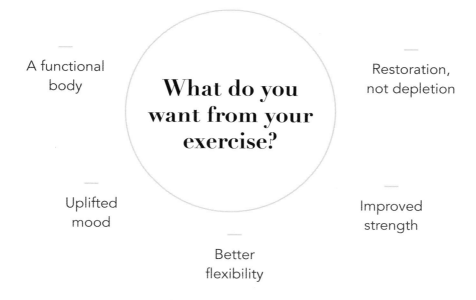

A functional body

Restoration, not depletion

What do you want from your exercise?

Uplifted mood

Improved strength

Better flexibility

What do you need from your body?

For your whole life, you want the ability to move and have the freedom to undertake the tasks you want and need to do. You do not want to rely on others to tie your shoelaces. You want to turn your head efficiently when you drive your car, to be able to carry your groceries and your children and grandchildren. Without a functional body, you can miss the joy, freedom and independence of these simple pleasures.

So what are good ways to achieve strength, flexibility and restoration from your movement? Some ideas include weights, yoga, pilates, t'ai chi, walking, swimming, playing with your children, stretching, taking the stairs instead of the lift, parking away from your destination and walking the rest of the way, gardening and farm work.

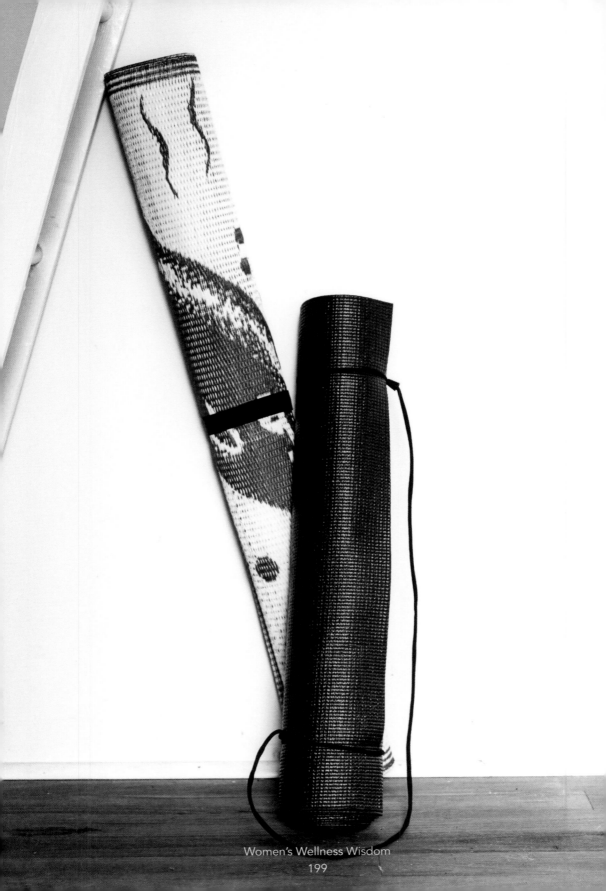

YOUR MOVEMENT

What movement types are you going to embrace to enhance your:

Strength

....

....

....

Flexibility

....

....

....

Restoration

....

....

....

....

You want to feel good after exercise, strong
and clear in your mind. Not depleted and spent.
Embrace movement patterns that serve your
needs and support your health, both now
and in the future.

Get up

IS SITTING SAPPING YOUR ENERGY?

Many adults spend too many of their waking hours sitting, with studies showing that some spend an enormous 11 hours per day on their bottoms. Those hours tend to be clocked up working at a desk job, commuting to and from work, watching television, or at the computer. Whatever the reason, research shows that too much sitting isn't good for health or energy.

Even if you are in the small proportion of people who do the recommended amount of at least 150 minutes of exercise per week (preferably a combination of walking — just being mobile — muscle-building resistance training, stretching and breath-focused restorative practices), you still need to move more regularly throughout the day. In other words, it is the sitting itself — not necessarily a lack of exercise — that adds to the undesirable impact on energy and specific health parameters. The amount of time spent sitting must decrease.

Physiologically, distinct effects are observed between prolonged sedentary time and too little physical activity. It seems likely that there is a unique physiology of sedentary time, within which biological processes that are distinct from traditionally-understood exercise physiology are operating. The groundbreaking work of Professor Marc Hamilton and colleagues provides a compelling body of evidence that the chronic, unbroken periods of muscular unloading associated with prolonged sedentary time may have deleterious biological consequences.

Physiologically, it has been suggested that the loss of local contractile stimulation induced through sitting leads to the suppression of skeletal muscle lipoprotein lipase (LPL) activity, which, put simply, is necessary for triglyceride (free fat in the blood) uptake and

recommended amount of at least

150

minutes
OF EXERCISE PER WEEK

HDL-cholesterol production, as well as reduced glucose uptake. You don't want to mess your LPL levels!

Hamilton's findings suggest that standing — which involves isometric contraction of the anti-gravity (postural) muscles and only low levels of energy expenditure — elicits skeletal muscle electrical changes as well as LPL changes. In other words, when we sit for too long, the body's ability to both utilize (burn) energy and create and experience energy is compromised. Think about it.

If you sit for four hours straight, do you bound up with energy or begin to droop over your desk and feel sluggish, lethargic and fatigued?

Typically, it's the latter.

LET'S MOVE IT

All of the health and poor energy risks that come from prolonged sitting can be reduced by taking regular breaks from sitting. Frequent, small amounts of movement have been shown to improve some blood markers for cardiovascular disease and type 2 diabetes. Plus, this has been shown to help clear some of the inflammatory products from the body and reduce the risk of weight gain that can occur through inflammatory processes.

Research has also shown that regular movement breaks across the day reduce back, neck and shoulder pain, plus boost mood, all factors that contribute to us experiencing better energy, both physically and emotionally.

To reap the health and energy benefits, it is best to get up from your desk every hour for about three to five minutes. You might like to set an alarm. Make it a gentle one or an inspiring, enlivening one, rather than one that grates your nerves, irritates you and activates the fight-or-flight response. Or find an app to remind you. Alternatively, you might like to get up each hour on the hour. You might like to walk up and down a flight of stairs a few times or walk the length of the office. Or get up to get yourself a glass of water from a location distant from your desk.

If you have a choice, you might choose to invest in a standing desk or create one from objects around your home or office.

Just be sure to stop sitting and to move every hour — and notice if more motion enhances your energy, productivity and feelings of wellness.

> It is best
> to get up
> **EVERY HOUR**
> for
> # 3 - 5
> minutes

FIVE WAYS TO MOVE

1 Take the stairs instead of a lift or an escalator.

2 Swap sitting meetings for walking meetings at work, using your phone to record the meeting. Spend five minutes at the end sitting and consolidating it all.

3 If you watch television, get up during commercial breaks and go for a walk around the house.

4 Engage in active travel to and from work or school, bike riding or walking, standing instead of sitting on public transport, and getting off a stop earlier so you have to walk further to your destination.

5 Swap sedentary family time for active family time. This might mean playing hide-and-seek or going to the park instead of watching television.

Remember it is what you do every day that impacts on your health and energy, not what you do sometimes. Just be conscious about how much you sit. Embrace more motion, preferably once each hour for three to five minutes. Your health, energy and ability to focus may all be enhanced in the process.

Why meditate?

HOW MEDITATION CAN HELP YOU THRIVE
IN TODAY'S BUSY WORLD

In today's world of deadlines, demands and a general desperation to create more time in our days, in order to get more done, it can be very easy to believe that there is no time to meditate. However, if that's how you feel, then you are the very person who needs to do it! We understand that for physical fitness we need to train our body — we can't just get up one day and do 50 chin-ups. The same is true for our mind: it requires a daily practice of "training", and meditation can be a part of that.

Meditation helps you to calm your mind, increases your focus and helps with time management — in other words, a short daily meditation practice will allow you to be more productive with the time you are given. A simple 10-15 minute breathing meditation can help you to activate your parasympathetic nervous system (which is responsible for rest and repair), reduce stress hormone levels, and find some calm.

For centuries, people have used meditation to move beyond the mind's often stress-inducing thoughts. Today, the variety of meditation techniques, traditions and technologies astound me, but the core of meditation remains the same: to bring peace to the mind and body and raise consciousness.

Meditation gives us the space to better understand our own mind. We can actively learn how to transform thoughts. It also teaches us how to overcome challenging mindsets and be more authentic. Some people are drawn to meditation at the recommendation of a health professional, to lower blood pressure and help with coping with stress and attaining restful sleep. Others find meditation as they are seeking transformation for the unhelpful emotions they are experiencing. While the purpose and intention of meditation depends on the meditator, anyone who meditates regularly will benefit mentally, emotionally, physically and spiritually.

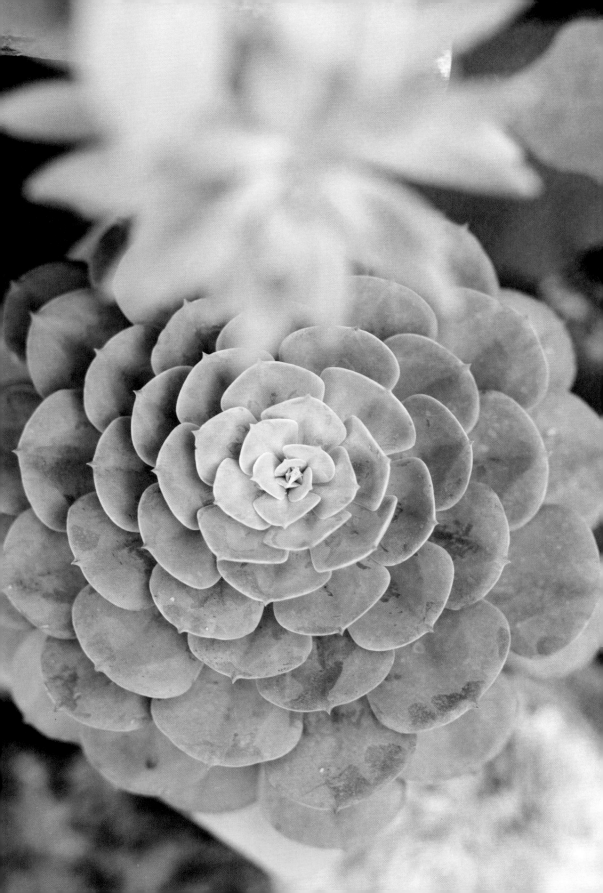

Something that has always fascinated me, though, is how easily meditation is not embraced at times, despite it being highly beneficial for someone. If the doctor tells a patient to take a pill twice a day with food to help them obtain a change with their health, almost everyone makes sure they do. Yet when health professionals suggest that a client meditates daily as it will give them the outcomes they are seeking, when you check in with them, many say they did it "sometimes, not every day, but occasionally". Really think about that, and keep in mind that when we say we don't have time for something, what we are really saying is that is not a priority for us. Just know that that is the case. It may be a practice you choose to explore down the track.

Regulation of high blood pressure (stress-induced)

Better clarity of thought or less mental clutter

the
BENEFITS
of regular
meditation
practice

Improved breathing (particularly with shallow-breathers)

Reduction in stress and anxious feelings

Improved sleep (typically more restful and deeper)

Ability to activate the parasympathetic nervous system

Try meditating early in the morning — perhaps before others in your household get up — as often this is the most peaceful time of the day, plus you are open to the newness of the day. Appreciate that it is an active process; it is hard to bring quiet to your mind and focus your attention to a single point. If you find your mind wanders, be kind to yourself and bring your focus back to your breath or a mantra.

Create the most nurturing environment you can, perhaps even light a candle. It is also important that you are comfortable: you don't have to sit cross-legged, and you can lie down or sit on a chair, whatever works for you.

I suggest you try

20 minutes

twice a day

Although many people try meditation at some point in their lives, not all stick with the practice for the long term. Read books on medtiation or listen to instructional CDs if this helps make it a regular practice. If you don't feel like it is something you can do by yourself, sign yourself up for a course and have someone guide you in finding the right style of meditation for you. I suggest you try 20 minutes twice a day. As with anything, though, often one size doesn't fit all. It can take a little bit of exploring to find the practice that works for you — but your mind, body and soul will love you for it! Keep in mind that you shower each day to wash the physical dirt off your body.

Meditation does that for your mind. And it brings you home to the truth of who you are.

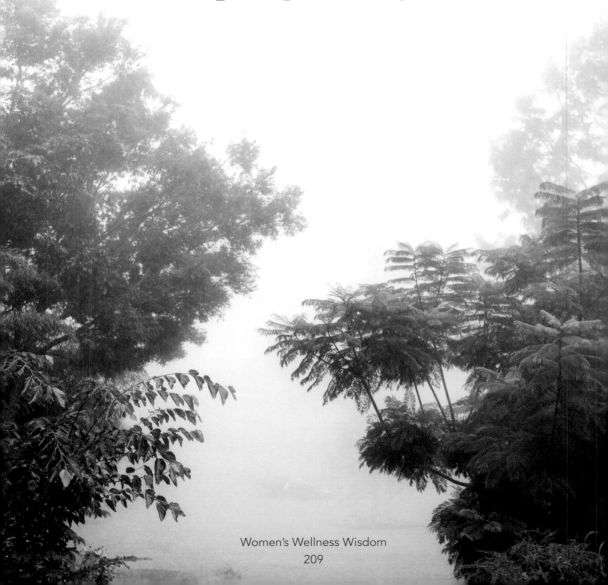

Relearn how to
BREATHE
diaphragmatically

BREATHE

The way you breathe has a powerful impact on your biochemistry, your ability to use body fat as a fuel, and your energy, predominantly via your nervous system.

The nervous system has many parts, one of which is the autonomic nervous system (ANS). The ANS has two branches: the sympathetic nervous system (SNS) and the parasympathetic nervous system (PNS). The SNS is the fight-or-flight response, while the PNS is the rest, digest, repair and reproduce arm of the nervous system. The challenge for so many people today is that they live in SNS dominance: they live constantly in the fight-or-flight response. Not that long ago (relative to the enormity of time humans have been on the planet), adrenalin, one of the main stress hormones that drives the SNS response, communicated to every cell in the body that our life was in danger. In modern times, we make adrenalin from the consumption of caffeine and the perception of pressure and urgency.

When your body perceives that your life is in danger, it has to supply you with a fast-burning fuel to get you out of that danger. The only two fuels for the human body are glucose and/or fat. Take a wild guess which is your fast-burning fuel? Glucose.

When you rely predominantly on glucose rather than body fat as your fuel, your clothes can become tighter and you live on an energy roller-coaster. It is like burning petrol on the flames of your energy fire. When your body can efficiently use fat as a fuel, your energy is robust and consistent across the day, with wood fuelling your energy fire. Activating the PNS plays a major role in the efficient utilization of body fat as a fuel, as your body feels "safe" to use it. Extending the length of your exhalation activates the PNS.

Become breath-aware for better energy.

How to breathe diaphragmatically

Find somewhere quiet to sit (floor, chair or lie down)

*Gently, place your hands on your belly and
look straight ahead or close your eyes*

*Take a long, slow inhale, breathing
through your nostrils*

*As you inhale, send the breath to your belly
and extend your belly with the inhale,
so that you can feel your hands gently
push forward with your belly*

*Imagine you have a balloon in your belly
and with each inhale you are inflating
that balloon*

*There is no need to hold your breath
here, just simply pause*

*Exhale slowly through your nostrils as
your belly shrinks back
toward your spine,
deflating the balloon*

Gently pause

*Begin to slowly inhale
again, extending
your belly as before*

Repeat this 10 times

It may feel uncomfortable initially as some of the muscles are not used to being used, but the more you practise this, the easier it gets, until you'll find yourself doing it automatically.

Breathing in this way is such beautiful nourishment for your nervous system, your pituitary gland, and your adrenals.

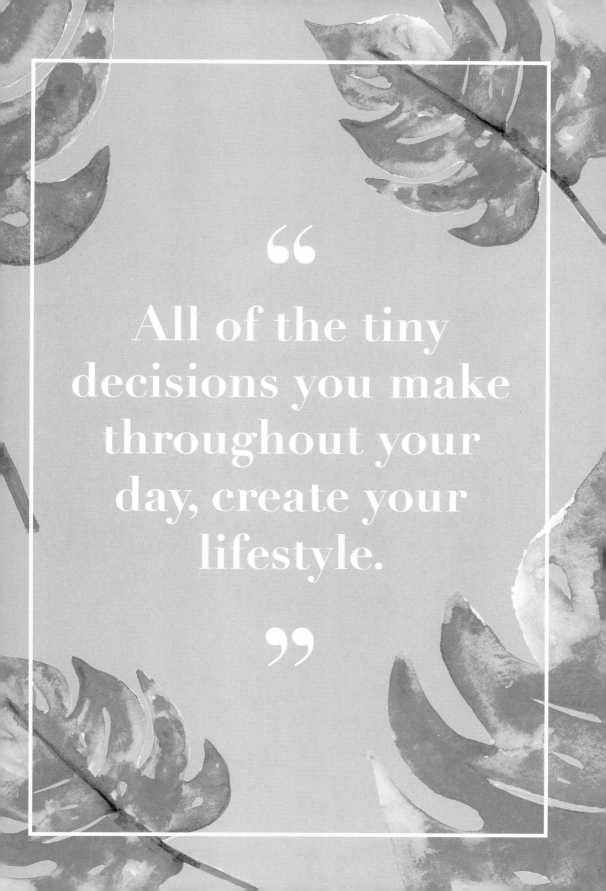

> 66
>
> All of the tiny decisions you make throughout your day, create your lifestyle.
>
> 99

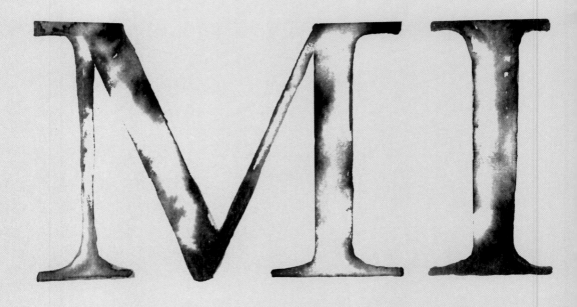

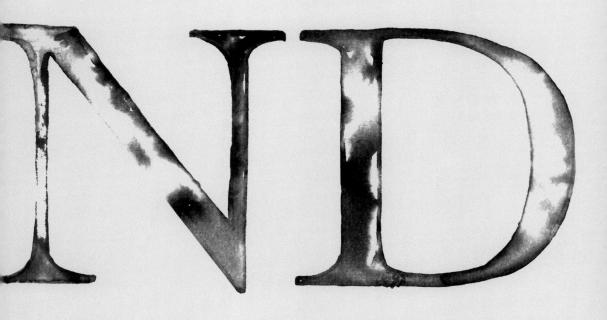

Your behaviour is the outer-most expression of your beliefs. The challenge is, most people aren't taught to examine what they believe about themselves, what occurs in their lives, or their choices, and instead they just don't really understand why they do what they do, even though they know what they know. Understanding that your mind creates meanings from what occurs every day, helps you to begin to unravel and gain deeper insights into your life and choices.

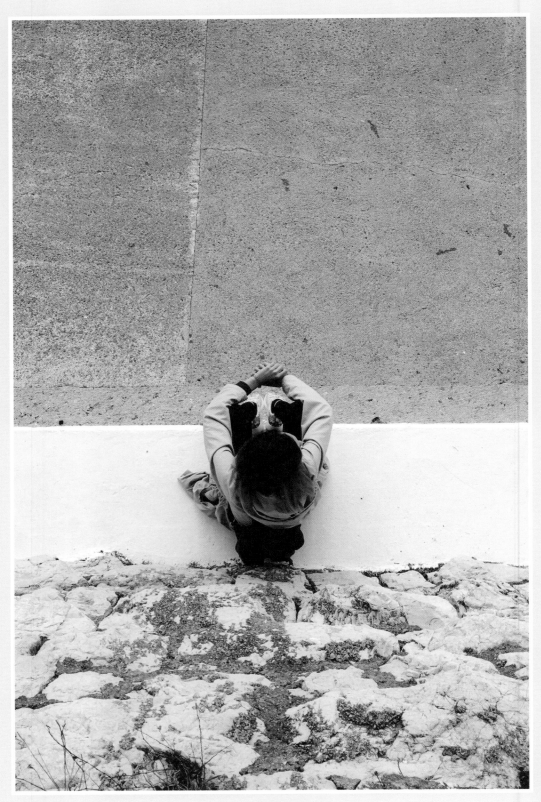

Emotional eating

WHAT DO YOU REALLY WANT?

When you have eaten and yet you still feel hungry, no food will fill the void for the type of hunger you feel. It is soul food you are looking for at this time, not food food. Yet the calorie equation, which too many people still falsely believe is the sole determinant of body shape and size, goes no way to examining this. It simply makes your hunger "wrong". You feel like your appetite must just be too big, and you worry that you will never lose weight or get your appetite under control, as usually the only strategy people have been given to lose weight is to eat less and move more. So you feel hopeless and feel that there must be something wrong with you, which only leads you to want to eat more to escape the feelings of your perceived worthlessness that you won't usually even be aware you are feeling.

A powerful strategy to apply in this state is what I have come to call my "What do I really want?" strategy. A page has been created for you at the end of this article to keep on hand, or you might prefer to create a page in a journal or a notebook that you divide into four columns with the headings:

- What do I want?
- What do I really want?
- How will having that make me feel?
- How else can I feel this emotion in a way that won't harm my health?

First, identify what do I want?

Ask yourself and then write down the answer. Let's say your response is "chocolate biscuits", but you have eaten not long ago, and you know you can't be physically hungry, so you ask the next question. What do I really want? Again, write your answer down. Let's say at first you still say "chocolate biscuits", but you keep asking yourself: what do I really want? And your response might be "a new bathroom", "a hug", "to be thinner", "a boyfriend" or "less financial stress".

But it is not really about having those things, because we are governed by how we feel. So you ask yourself the next question: How will having that make me feel? And your answer might be "happy", "appreciated", "loved", "relieved" or "successful", for example.

Then you follow that up with the final question: How else can I feel this emotion in a way that won't harm my health? And write down your answers. You might say "dance around the house", "read", "watch my children sleep", "phone a friend" or "do something for someone else that makes them feel appreciated", as examples.

Get in touch with what you really want to feel, and do the things that lead you to feel this way far more often. Then observe how your desire for extra food after you have eaten begins to fall away. You can also use this strategy if you make poor-quality food choices, even though you know better. You might not understand why you always go for a packet of chips for dinner instead of eating a more nourishing meal.

Exploring how you really want to feel, and finding ways to do this other than consuming food, can be your gateway to making nourishing food choices effortless.

You can begin to do this, using the worksheet over the page.

> When you have eaten and yet you still feel hungry, no food will fill the void for the type of hunger you feel. It is soul food you are looking for at this time, not food food.

What do you really want?

1 WHAT DO I WANT?

e.g. chocolate biscuits

....

....

....

....

....

....

....

....

....

....

....

2 WHAT DO I REALLY WANT?

e.g. a hug

....

....

....

....

....

....

....

....

....

....

....

3 HOW WOULD HAVING THAT MAKE ME FEEL?

e.g. loved and appreciated

4 HOW ELSE CAN I EXPERIENCE THAT FEELING?

e.g. write an old friend a letter telling her how much I appreciate her

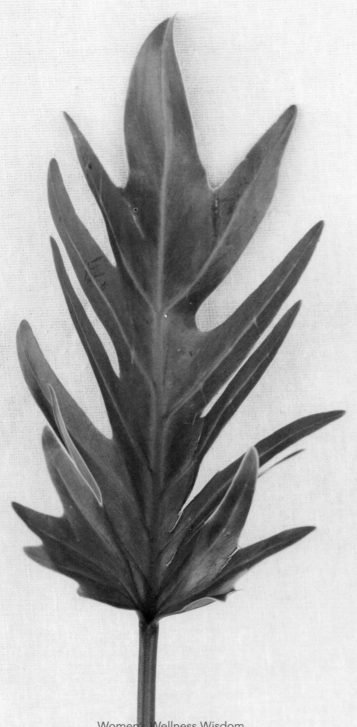

Not enoughness

The belief that you are not, and don't have enough might manifest in unkind behaviour towards the people you actually love. It may manifest as a desperate feeling for more — more of anything or anyone — which might show up in your life as eating too much, spending beyond your means, or frequent, brief intimate encounters. A belief that you don't have enough will make you utterly blind to, and entirely callous about, those who have less, because you believe that you are one of them. When you are caught in a trance of deficiency, your task, your only task, is to do whatever it takes to get more. If fortune throws a significant amount of money in your lap, you won't see it. You will find a way to make it disappear so that the world you live in will be congruent with your beliefs. With decades of experiments examining everything from the efficacy of wrinkle creams to observations on car colours, scientists have discovered that we don't believe what we see, rather we see what we believe.

Until you are willing to name your beliefs — whether because circumstances force your hand, or because you wake up to the pain of seeing through shattered lenses, or because you are sick of living your life in a great big rush and the subsequent health consequences — you will continue to act on your self-created version of reality. This is why a person who believes that people can't be trusted will see "evidence" of this everywhere, and they will miss noticing all of the people who can be trusted. It is why lottery winners tend to blow through their cash and end up broke: even with millions, they believe they are poor, and actions always conform to beliefs. Unless you name your beliefs, you will continue to believe that your version of reality is the way that it is, not the way that you choose it to be based on your beliefs. Naming beliefs and exploring the feelings that arise is an ongoing, exciting, heart-opening process.

There are times when rushing serves a brilliant purpose, and when it is short-lived there is no problem for our physical and emotional health. We cope without a hitch. But when you live in that state day after day, year after year, it can take an immense toll on your health. When I work with women and can see that rushing is at the heart of the health problems they have come to see me about, they firstly either deny that they are stressed (despite their blood tests showing that they are) and tell me that this is just how their life is, or they agree to slow down ("Funny you say that: my mother is always telling me to slow down," they'll say), but they don't. Nothing about their lifestyle changes. And the best diet in the world, the best supplements, or the best exercise plan, won't even touch the sides when your sympathetic nervous system (SNS) is always dominant. And to allow your parasympathetic nervous system (the rest and digest arm) to do its vital work, you first need to understand what SNS dominance is actually doing to you, and therefore why you need to change, and then, secondly, you need to explore your emotional landscape to see why you feel the need to do everything with urgency.

You have very ancient hormonal mechanisms in action inside your body that believe they know better than you when it comes to your survival. Your body can be your biggest teacher if you learn how to decipher the messages it is communicating to you. And your behaviours, extra body fat or an unjustified panicked perception of life are sometimes simply vehicles of communication, doing their best to remind you to rest the part of you that is weary, and awaken the part of you that is asleep. And mostly the part of women that has gone to sleep is our belief, our deep knowing of how precious we are and that we deserve nothing but the best care, the utmost of kindness and nurturing, and nourishment for our body, mind, and soul; gifts we can choose to give ourselves every single day.

And for the mothers, in particular, the women for whom guilt has become a way of life, I ask you to remember this sentiment: you are the best mother your child will ever have. You are their barometer and their compass in this world. And every single child thinks that their mother is absolutely wonderful.

> ## We don't believe what we see, rather we see what we believe.

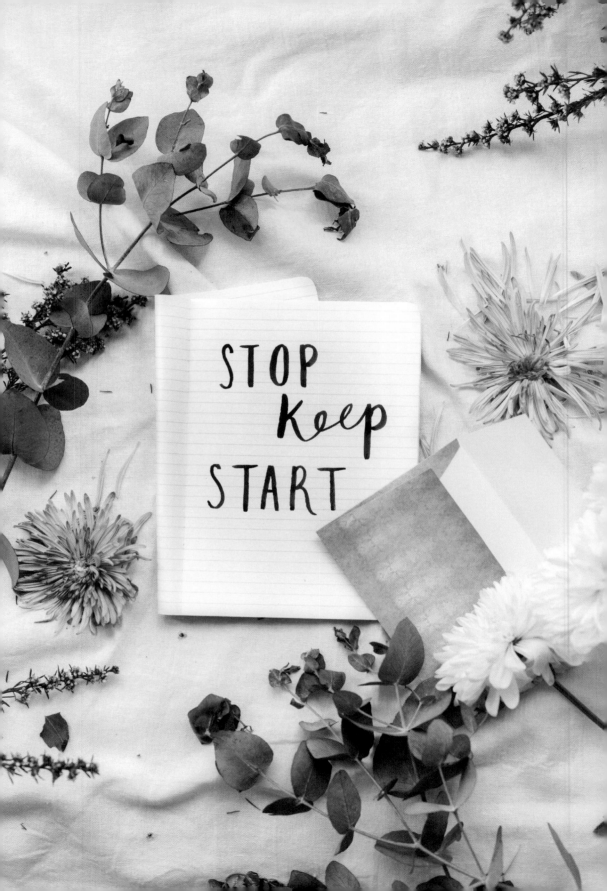

24 hours?

If you feel that having too much to do is contributing to your stress levels, then another useful strategy you might like to adopt is known as Stop. Keep. Start.

Here, we have drawn up columns with each of those words as a heading. Take some time to fill in some items in each column, prompting yourself with the following questions:

What am I going to stop doing?

What am I going to keep doing?

What am I going to start doing?

STOP	KEEP	START

You can use the suggestions on these pages to help you begin.

Here is a sample:

STOP:

I am going to stop getting caught up in gossip, as it is exhausting.

KEEP:

I am going to keep eating a nourishing breakfast every day.

START:

I am going to start walking four days out of seven for the next two weeks, starting tomorrow morning at 6am.

Stop, keep and start goals can make change fun, manageable and suitable for your lifestyle. While I was writing *Exhausted to Energized*, I read a blog post written by the brilliant Danielle LaPorte, and it inspired me to ask people from all walks of life about things they had stopped, started or continued doing that had really served them, and particularly their energy, in any area of life.

Here are some of the answers that I especially enjoyed from many different people, and in their own words:

- started drinking warm lemon water first thing in the morning. It has really helped my digestion and skin

- got black-out curtains for my bedroom and removed anything that blinked or flashed. Welcome circadian rhythm contentment!

- scheduled a weekly bush walk with a girlfriend. It gets me into Nature, and we are happy walking in silence or chatting. I feel so much better after I do this each week, even though before I go I never feel like I have the time

- started doing Stillness Through Movement classes (a form of restorative yoga) twice a week. Literally. Changed. My. Life. And I don't say that lightly

- started a computer course at my local technical college. I am 74 years old, but I was missing out seeing my family on their Facebook page, not being able to use a computer. Now I feel more connected to them because I can use the computer and see their photographs. And I know how to type them a message now

- went gluten-free

- set up my office at home as if it is a real office, a real room, worthy of lovely treasures, rather than the "spare room made in to an office". I feel organized and less stressed, and I look forward to going in there now

- found the courage to admit to my boss that I don't like managing people, and therefore I am not excellent at managing people. Thankfully, she changed my role to not manage people, and I feel like I have a new life!

- started getting up at 5am each morning and having an hour to myself

- started watching my children sleep (about an hour after they fall asleep) for 10 minutes each evening. Seeing them so peaceful makes me feel so calm before I get more done in the evening. I feel like I approach my nightly tasks with a different attitude after I've watched them sleeping

- continued getting up at 5am, and I meditate, give thanks for my life, read (learn) and watch the sun rise each morning. It changed my life and I don't plan on ever changing this ritual. I'm only sorry I didn't start doing this until I was 46

- started cleaning out my clothes cupboard every six months, and I give what I haven't worn in the last chunk of time to a charity shop so they can sell it and make money

- stopped responding to text messages immediately just because they were text messages. Remember when not that much was urgent? This gives me such a sense of freedom

- started taking voice lessons. It changed the way I breathe. And when I changed the way I regularly breathe, my posture and presence and hence my effectiveness and happiness all shifted in the most powerful way

- started meditating daily. No. Matter. What.

- started and have continued to become harder to get hold of [this person was very well known in the health and healing world] so I could have more spaciousness and ease in my life. I decided that if it interfered with me being home when my daughter gets home from school, then I'm a no, thank you

- my son had been diagnosed with a mental health disorder. He loves music. So we got him a guitar and then went through guitar teachers until we found the one who said, "Forget scales. What song do you want to learn to play today?" I cannot tell you the truly wonderful impact this has had on our lives

- I started going to bed before midnight. That danger zone between 11.30pm and midnight — when I get my second wind of the day... I stopped pushing through that to do more emails or start another task — and I shut it all down. If I'm in bed before midnight, I fall asleep straight away. If I pass the warning zone and stay up, I fire up again and it takes longer to unwind for sleep. Anything I think I need to do after 11.30pm can wait until the morning. What I do (for home or work) is not more important than my sleep. No one will actually die if I don't start a new pile of emails at 11.30pm

Your turn.

HOW WOULD YOU ANSWER THE QUESTIONS:

What am I going to STOP doing?

....

....

....

....

....

What am I going to KEEP doing?

....

....

....

....

....

What am I going to START doing?

....

....

....

....

....

....

....

The results for your health and energy may astonish you.

Resourceful questions

HAVE YOU EVER HEARD THE SAYING "QUESTIONS ARE THE ANSWERS"?

Have you pondered this long enough to experience the truth in it? Whenever you ask your brain a question, it will always give you an answer. Ask a lousy-quality question, and you will usually get a lousy answer.

Perhaps you find yourself always asking, "Why does this always happen to me?" Your brain will usually come up with a rather insulting response to this, simply reiterating your fears that you aren't good enough the way you are. If you change that question to "Why is this happening for me?" your brain will immediately look for the way this situation is helping you.

A question-based concept that I have witnessed has benefited many is one known as a "primary question". This is a question we silently, usually unknowingly, subconsciously ask ourselves before we do or decide anything. And I mean anything. And it determines what we consistently notice and experience in life. It was usually created when we were very young, and it is not something we consciously chose, but rather it formed as a result of a challenge we faced. We originally created it to help keep ourself safe, usually from emotional pain.

Here's a common example. You may be familiar with the foundational idea that "what you focus on, you feel" and "what you focus on, you get more of". In other words, whatever filter we apply to a given situation will shape our experience of that situation. Let's imagine, for instance, that someone has a history of what they perceive to be "failed" relationships. As a result of how they view their history, they might approach any new relationship asking themselves, "Is this relationship going to fail, too?" This question will tend to create a self-fulfilling prophecy, as this person will predominantly focus on whatever might go wrong with their new partner, rather than pay attention to what might be going well and what they could do to improve areas that they or the other person find challenging.

Your primary question is cross-contextual — meaning it doesn't only come into play in one area of your life (such as relationships) — and is most noticeable in stressful situations. Going back to the example above, we could extrapolate that the person might apply the "failure" filter to a number of contexts other than intimate relationships. That person's underlying primary question in life may be "Am I going to fail?" Although a number of other factors come into play as well, this primary question will undoubtedly have an impact on the course of action the person will choose when presented with what they might perceive as a stress-inducing opportunity, such as a promotion at work. If they strongly value change and adventure, they might still choose to accept the promotion despite their fear of failure. However, if they value certainty and security instead, they will be more likely to stay within their comfort zone and, as a result, are more likely to decline an offer that would otherwise drive them to face their fear. You need to understand the power of this: to this person, to feel like a failure is almost like death.

What could be an alternative primary question such a person might choose to ask themselves in order to achieve more of what they want? Or to stop fear ruling their choices? As a general rule, the best types of questions are solution-focused "how" and "what" questions that begin with the end in mind. Notice what comes up for you when you ask yourself, "How could I succeed?" or "What can I do to make this work?" Now compare it with what comes up when you ask closed "yes/no" questions or justification-prone "why" questions, like: "Am I going to fail?" or "Why do I keep failing?"

Another common example of a primary question I have heard over the years is "How can I ensure that I never let anyone down?" Can you hear how this presupposes that this person is going to disappoint someone? Can you actually disappoint someone? No. Their response to you is based on their life up until now. Only they can choose how they respond. For someone to feel disappointed in you, they will have had expectations, and those will be based on them, not you. Someone who never wants to let anyone down feels immense guilt in their daily life. They are people who can't usually tell you what they want or need; their response to "What do you need?" is usually "for my friends and family to be happy and healthy". They are highly adapted at focusing on what others need, not on their own needs. They are kind people. Yet there is immense fear there also. They walk on eggshells around anyone who behaves with more intensity than they do. And they struggle to make decisions, as they don't know what they want. On some level they do, but they can't access it, they can't see it. Guilt, as a result of their anticipation of letting others down, permeates and stifles them in every situation.

For these people, a better question to ask is one that presupposes that love or caring is present. For example, "How can I bring even more love and appreciation to this situation?" will offer someone a very different answer from "How can I ensure that I never let anyone down?"

Ask a different question and you will get a different answer. The quality of your life depends enormously on the quality of the questions you ask yourself.

Here are some tips to help you to find out what your primary question might be — and to help you replace it with a more supportive one, if needs be.

In this process, it is important to remain flexible and open: the point is not to find the absolute "perfect" question, but to become aware of disempowering thinking patterns so that you can replace them with more resourceful ones that bring you closer to what you actually want.

Think of a specific time in your personal life where you felt stuck. What were you focusing on? What main question might you have been asking yourself?

....

....

....

....

....

....

Now think of a specific situation in the context of work where you felt stuck. What were you focusing on? Again, what main question might you have been asking yourself?

....

....

....

....

....

See if you can find the common denominator between both questions and come up with a more open and solution-focused "how" or "what" type of question that you know would have supported you better. Make sure it presupposes that something you value (love, appreciation, or success, for example) is present. For example "How can I bring even more love and appreciation to this situation?"

....

....

....

....

....

In the future, whenever you catch yourself stuck in a situation, take a moment to notice what you are focusing on, enquire within about what question you might be asking yourself, and refocus your experience by asking the new question you have come up with — or with any other solution-focused question you can think of in the moment. Repeat this process time and time again until it becomes a new habit.

You will notice that your old primary question runs the show the more stressful a situation is for you. Be patient with yourself about this, and bring curiosity to these scenarios, never judgement of yourself or others. You have never walked in anyone else's shoes, just as they have no idea what it is like to be you. I have witnessed first-hand how asking better-quality questions can literally change the path of your life.

Over to you. What is your primary question? And what new, more empowering question can you now ask instead?

"

The difference between how you
are and how you want to be is in
the actions you take, which are
created by the thoughts you think,
fostered by your perception of
how things are and how you are,
behind which are your beliefs.

Changing the belief,
changes the actions.

"

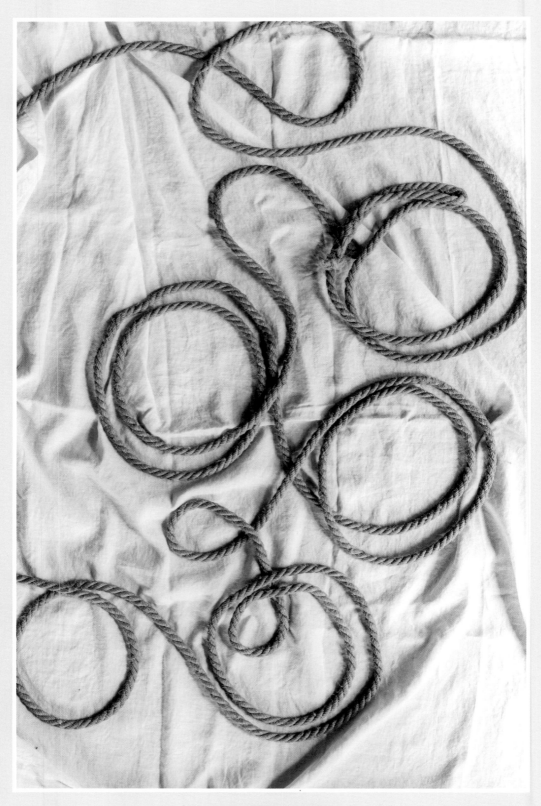

Women's Wellness Wisdom

Open loops

HOW TO CLOSE THEM

When I wrote my book *Exhausted to Energized*, one of the topics I discussed that has become a talking point since is that of "open loops". Or you might prefer to think of them as "open tabs". Consider this analogy. We all know that, the more programs we have open and the more things we are asking our computer or smart phone to do, the more it slows down and the more battery it burns. Twenty-seven open tabs of web pages, spreadsheets, documents and presentations, photo editing, movie playing, music, software updates... Our mind can feel very much the same. The more topics you have open and unresolved, the bigger the drain on your mind power and energy, from all of these open loops.

How many times across a day, a week, a month, a year, decades even, do tasks or situations open up, yet they are never resolved, finalized or closed? How many emails do you read that you don't immediately reply to, and they hang in your mind and add to your task load of what's not yet done? It is as if you walk around each day with so many tabs open — like websites sitting open on your computer screen — that you never feel like you have got it all handled. You never feel like you can rest. So you don't, not properly, even if you try. Plus, you might judge yourself for this. You might subconsciously tell yourself that you are a failure for not getting more done. Or that you are lazy, or hopeless or a fraud. Yet you may be completely unaware that you are judging yourself in this way.

Do you think these statements to and about yourself energize and uplift you, and empower you to take care of what's on your plate? Unlikely. Usually such harsh self-talk zaps the wind from your sails, and you live most days perceiving that you are proving yourself right — that you don't get enough done in a day, you procrastinate, and then the judgement begins all over again (if it ever paused) — and this depletes your energy further. Significantly.

You could consider that these open-loop scenarios offer you endless opportunities to experience amazing things in life. But most people see them as an utterly exhausting pile of stuff that they wish they could hand over to someone else.

The solutions? Scheduling your time.

Following through on what you say you will do. Delegating, if you are in a position to do this. Accept, as Oprah famously said, that you need to "Do what you have to do, until you can do what you want to do." When you fight with what is, when you battle with the ways things are, you suffer. So schedule what you will complete today and start closing some of those loops.

Keep an eye out for open loops. They can be a major drain on your health and energy without you being aware that they are doing so.

Further to this concept, while I was writing *Exhausted to Energized* I met with and interviewed people from all walks of life, and I also continued to read widely. With the open loops concept in my mind, I wanted to know how some of the busiest people in the world manage their time and get so much done!

The concept of time management was discussed a great deal with many people. I share a condensed version of that with you here.

You can try closing some loops using these four steps, which are employed by many busy people I know:

1 Identify and capture in writing everything that is open in your mind, that you are thinking about that needs resolution.

2 Organize these into simple headings that relate the importance of each task and its urgency; cluster the topics in categories.

3 Schedule times to consider, reflect, decide and execute the idea.

4 If it is not time to perform step 3 on the task or idea yet, then just know you have captured it and the time will come for you to schedule it.

Your "NO" muscle

DO YOU NEED TO FLEX IT MORE FREQUENTLY?

You are busy with what you say yes to.

There are plenty of people who find saying "no" a breeze, yet for others, it feels like an impossible task.

Do you need to flex your "no" muscles more regularly? If it's not a "hell yes!" then maybe it needs to be a "no"? If you are a people pleaser in your nature, then you will find it hard to say no and you may be exhausted from trying to appear stronger than you feel. You will find it easier to say no, however, if you focus on what you are giving the other person when you say no – growth, the opportunity to develop other resources, flexibility, an expanded view of the world, or a more authentic friendship, for example.

Being busy can lead us to use the language "I don't have time". Instead, try saying, "That's just not a priority for me at the moment" and see how that feels. This can help you decipher what you really want to say yes to, what your priorities are, and for many people today, this alone helps them to experience a greater sense of spaciousness, more calm, cultivate better personal energy and experience a greater level of wellness.

Take some time to reflect on what areas of your life, or whom, you find it hard to say "no" to.

....

....

....

....

....

....

Then ask yourself "What am I afraid will occur if I say no?" Begin to explore what this is really about.

....

....

....

....

....

....

....

....

....

....

....

....

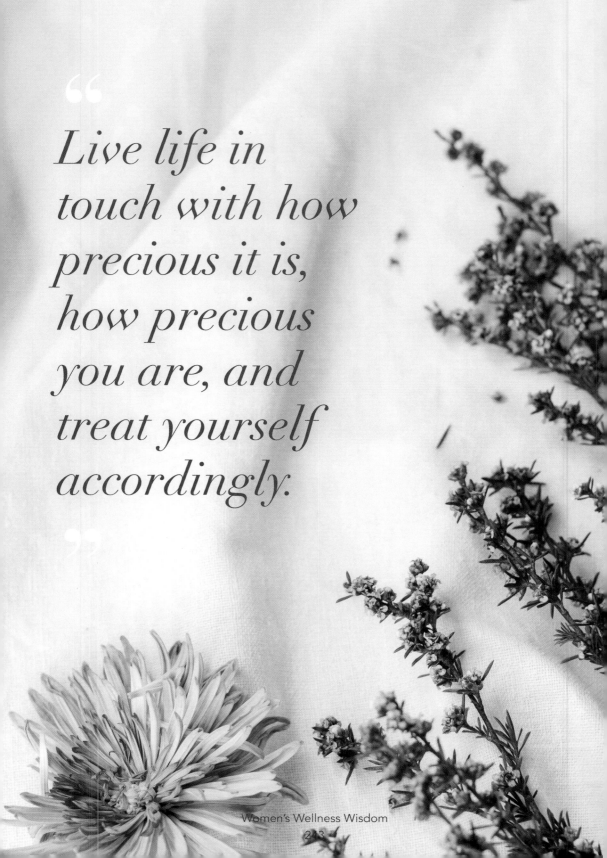

" *Live life in touch with how precious it is, how precious you are, and treat yourself accordingly.* "

Meaning maker

HOW *"GO AND GET CHANGED"* STARTED AN EATING DISORDER

Having worked with thousands of patients over the years who have experienced disordered eating in its many forms, I wanted to share a story with you, one that shows a psychological process that we all do to ourselves, and that can present in our lives in so many different ways. In this case, it was a straightforward request ("go and get changed") that had a major impact.

Imagine a whiteboard in front of you. Imagine I draw on it a big circle, and in that circle I write what happened, and then beside that circle I draw another circle and in that circle I write meaning. What we do is we merge the "what happened" with the "meaning", and then we live our lives as if the meaning is what actually happened.

The family in this story consisted of mum, dad and two daughters, aged 14 and eight. One day, Dad phoned home near the end of the day and suggested that he meet the three of them at a restaurant for dinner. So mum tells the girls that this is what is happening, and asks them to go and get changed, ready to meet dad and have dinner. The 14-year-old appears later wearing a crop-top, abdomen exposed. Mum says: "You need to go and get changed." A few days later, Mum overhears Ms 14 talking on the phone to one of her friends, saying, "Well, my mum thinks I'm fat." After Ms 14 gets off the phone, mum approaches Ms 14 and asks her why she said that to her friend, to which Ms 14 replies, "Because you said it the other day." Mum says that she did not say that, and that she would never say that. She says that she knows she didn't say it because she doesn't even believe it; in fact, the opposite is true, and she is actually worried that Ms 14 is too thin. Mum finishes with the question: "When do you think I said this?" Ms 14 replies: "The other day when you told me to go and get changed before we met Dad for dinner."

So in the circle with the words "what happened" I would now write: Mum told me to go and get changed. In the circle with the word "meaning" in it, I would now write: Mum thinks I'm fat. Had mum not overheard Ms 14 on the phone, Ms 14 would have carried that belief (that her mother thinks she is fat) into her future years. For how long? Who knows? But this is one way an eating disorder can be created. Not through malice or harshness, or through it being anyone's fault. Just because our brain is set up to merge what happens with the meanings we create about what happened. It is not a conscious process. You don't stand there in contemplation when mum says "go and get changed" and wonder what meaning you need to create from her words. It all occurs in your nervous system in a split second. And then you live your life looking for evidence of your new belief. Again, completely unaware that you now do this. And it impacts on every choice you make. We need to "un-merge" the "what happened" from the "meaning".

In my TEDx talk and most of my books and events, I talk a lot about the theme of "not-enoughness". It can feel like a never-ending tangle of string. All you need to begin, though, is an awareness of these patterns and a desire to live in another way, with new tools and strategies and a new level of self-care and appreciation for yourself and for life. When you judge (for we all do), whether yourself or another person, simply notice that you did so, and work out why. For inside those "whys" there is so much freedom and spaciousness.

If you are someone who, in your heart of heart, knows they don't eat enough, explore with kindness and curiosity whose love and attention you desperately want. And ask yourself: What would my heart have me do? Starve? No. What would courage have me do? Speak. Ask for help. Ask for a hug. It is never about the food or the lack of it. It is about how you perceive how not eating enough makes you feel. But getting to feel the feeling you want to feel by depriving yourself of nourishment hurts your health and impacts on those around you. It is time to find other ways to feel the feelings that you want to feel, without hurting your health. Often the root, as it is for so many situations, is a desire to feel loved. And once you find your path, you will naturally guide others to do the same. Now that's inspiring.

MEANING MAKER

Notice how quickly "your interpretation" is generated after the "what happened" occurs. Notice how much bigger "your interpretation" feels compared to the "what happened". We then merge the two and the "meaning" is created. We then take that meaning into the future and see "evidence" of it everywhere. And we miss all of the examples of how the story we created isn't true.

WHAT HAPPENED?

YOUR INTERPRETATION

MEANING YOU CREATED

Dear Beautiful Girl,

Don't settle for a life that you live in the cloud of false belief that you aren't beautiful. Don't let it take until your life is about to end before you feel deep in your heart what you have always known — that you are, and have always been, beautiful. Live your life now, awake, and lit-up with that knowing, impacting the lives of others with your light.

What is your word? What is the word written in gorgeous handwriting across your heart? What gift do you bring to every situation when you really show up? Name it. Is it "fun", "kindness", "joker" or "quiet observer who then shares her golden insights" (more than one word, I know!)? Or is it "magician", "angel", "wonder", "fabulousness" or "optimist"? Never underestimate the power you bring, the difference you make, and the gift you are to this world.

Never stop believing. Never stop believing in your own radiance, even if you feel others have urged you to dim your own light. You don't stop believing in the sun when the moon comes out. You don't stop believing in the moon when the clouds pass over her face. You may have a moment when you judge yourself harshly. You may have days or — hopefully not — weeks when you feel anything but beautiful. But never stop believing in your beauty, even if it momentarily disappears from your own view, because of choices you have made. You are not your behaviour. You need to take responsibility for your behaviour, but you are not it. We usually behave poorly when we perceive (notice that I say "perceive") that we have lost, or may lose, love or acceptance, or if we perceive that we have failed. But there is no failure. It's all just feedback.

Be just like the sun that shines its light upon the world. Remember that you, too, light up the world with your very presence. Beauty is a light in your heart, and it doesn't just light up your own gorgeous face; it lights up the whole world. For when we let our own light shine, we give others permission to do the same. Open your eyes wide and see the wonder in the world. Open your eyes wide, knowing that there is wonder in your heart, and marvel at the wonder that you are.

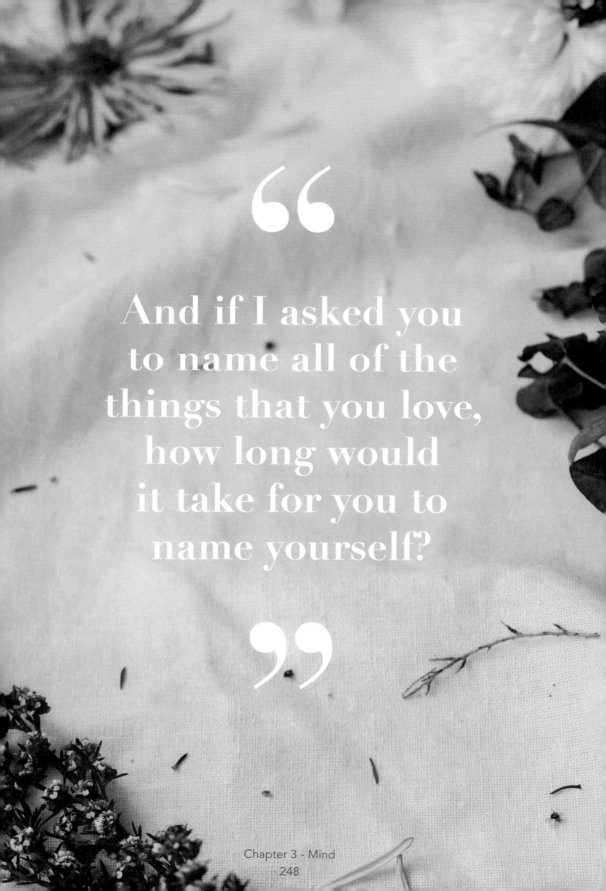

"

And if I asked you
to name all of the
things that you love,
how long would
it take for you to
name yourself?

"

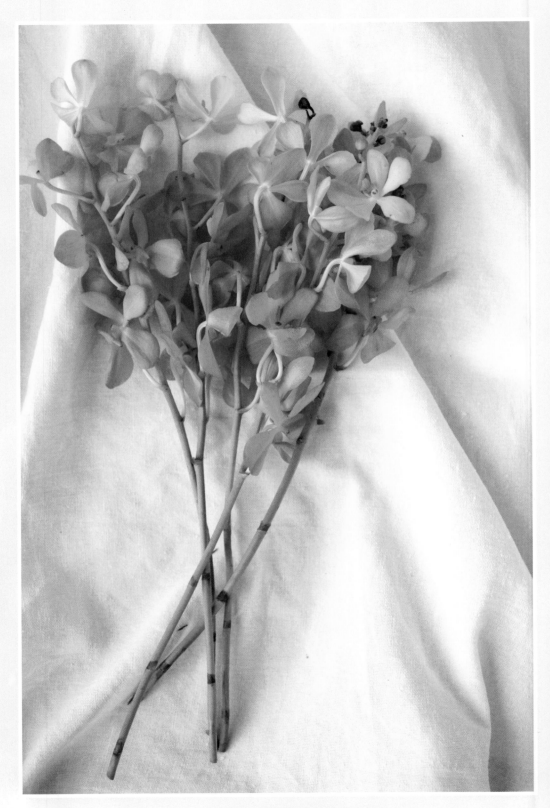

Women's Wellness Wisdom

A 'no' uttered from the deepest conviction is better than a 'yes' merely uttered to please, or worse, to avoid trouble.

Mahatma Gandhi

Contribution

LIFT OTHERS, LIFT YOURSELF

Often when we feel like the weight of the world is on our shoulders, making a difference in the lives of others can be the last thing on our mind. Yet it is often just the remedy you need. When we feel unhappy, we are almost always focused on ourselves, and when we contribute to the lives of others it shifts our focus. What you focus on is what you feel. And when you give to others, you receive so much in return. The joy of giving is such a win-win, for the giver and the receiver.

Here are some ideas that you might like to do randomly, or make a part of your life on a regular basis.

Pick up any litter you see.

Write a letter or send a card to someone you haven't spoken to in a while.

Cook and deliver dinner to an elderly neighbour or to a busy family who would really appreciate it.

Donate money to a charity making a difference. For example, in our office, we have all sorts of challenges, and the winning prize is $50 given to the Fred Hollows Foundation – they can restore someone's sight for $25.

Give money, a warm drink or a warm jumper to someone who is without a home at the moment.

Volunteer for an organization that helps people in need.

Volunteer at an animal shelter, as many are non-profit and and therefore welcome volunteers to help take care of animals, keep facilities clean and work with the public.

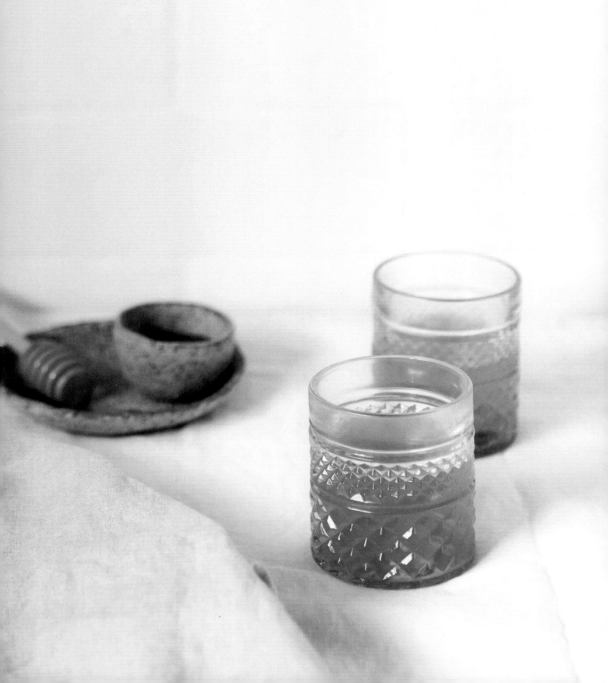

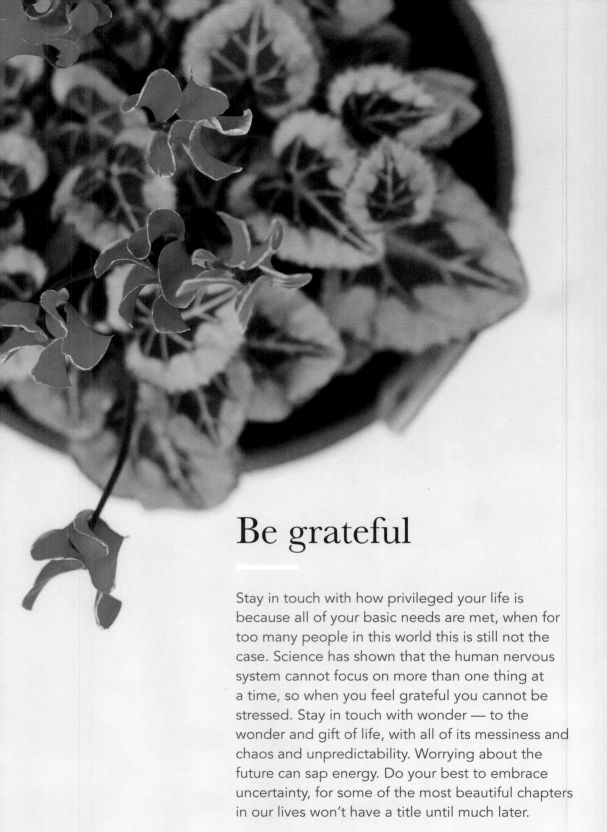

Be grateful

Stay in touch with how privileged your life is because all of your basic needs are met, when for too many people in this world this is still not the case. Science has shown that the human nervous system cannot focus on more than one thing at a time, so when you feel grateful you cannot be stressed. Stay in touch with wonder — to the wonder and gift of life, with all of its messiness and chaos and unpredictability. Worrying about the future can sap energy. Do your best to embrace uncertainty, for some of the most beautiful chapters in our lives won't have a title until much later.

"

Do your best
to embrace
uncertainty, for
some of the most
beautiful chapters
in our lives won't
have a title until
much later.

"

Let yourself have what you already have

———

Even if it is right in front of you every day, and you don't let yourself have it — which means noticing it, taking it in, allowing yourself the pleasure of it — it is never yours.

It never becomes part of the ground of goodness on which you can live, and this, the essence of this, forms so much of our foundation of health and energy that isn't really discussed.

If you don't let yourself have an amazing sunset, a cool evening breeze on your face after a hot day, a majestic view, then what else are you denying yourself?

Why not let yourself have what you already have?

I have read that when people who are dying are asked what they will miss the most, they say, *"The ordinary things. The smell in the air just before rain. The feeling of my dog's fur under my hands. My partner's face. A freshly cut lemon. The night sky."*

We have those now. Let yourself have what you already have. It's what joy is all about and joy gives us an irreplaceable depth of energy.

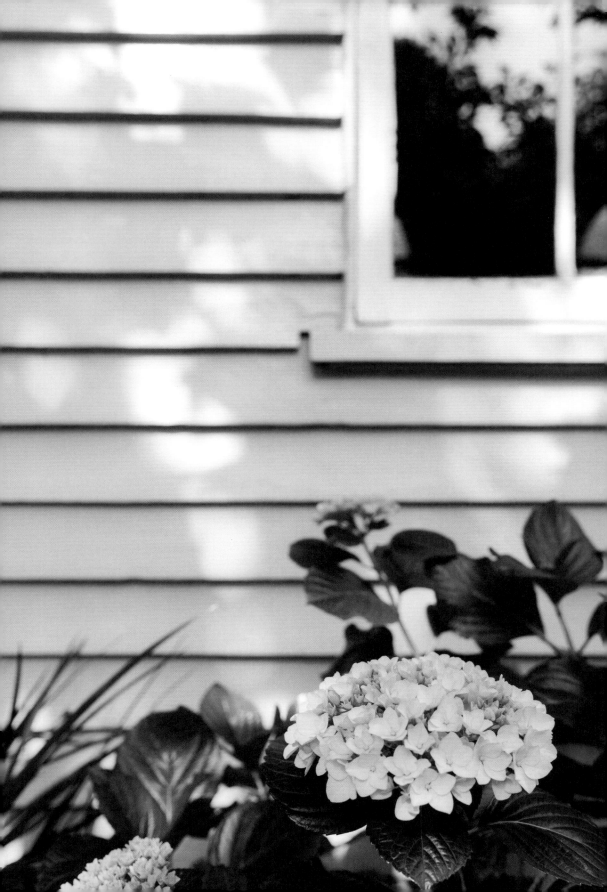

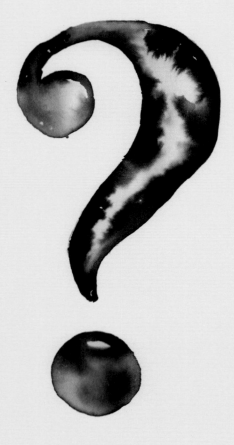

Women's Wellness Wisdom

Giving things up

OR BLIND TO THEIR PURPOSE?

In psychology, it is taught that dysfunctional behaviour in children is about unmet needs. I can't tell you how many young girls and boys I have met who have resorted to starving themselves, bingeing, stealing, cutting themselves, lying, bullying, allowing themselves to be victimized, or acting out in some way in a desperate attempt to meet an underlying emotional need.

So if this is true of children, it is likely to be true of adults as well, given that many people live emotionally frozen from some point in the past, in some ways, having not emotionally matured beyond a stressful time in their lives. I hear about it daily. As adults, we can function as part of normal society, but behind closed doors where we get triggered — which will show up as an intense emotional reaction to something someone says or to something that occurs — we resort to the behaviour we displayed around the age of the emotional wounding. Much dysfunctional behaviour with food stems from people trying to avoid feeling the emotional pain of the past. Yet they are usually out of touch with the fact that this is what they are doing.

When all we do is try to educate people to change how they eat (too much food, not enough food, too much poor-quality food when they know better), and not the why, their feelings are further ignored. They can't stick to a "diet" — which will be seen as deprivation, and in some cases starvation, by the person on the receiving end of the instruction — for the very reason that they have been using food to numb their pain. Moreover, no sustained change ever occurs from a place of deprivation and starvation. It always begins with kindness. And I don't use the word "always" in that sentence without careful consideration.

If you take away the mechanism someone has been using to cope for five or 50 years, and don't replace it with anything, or don't get to the heart of the base issue and resolve it, they will return to the food or find another way — another obsession or addiction — to numb their pain. When they do this, they feel like a failure, like they are still not good enough, like they are hopeless, pathetic, that they have no willpower. Many people start using food to numb their pain as children or in their teenage years. For some, it is during or after a challenging relationship in adulthood. They have blanketed their feelings so heavily that they can't see that they eat to avoid experiencing emotions they don't want to feel.

When food is set up to be about numbers (counting calories, for example) and strict rules, you set up people who eat emotionally to not be able to eat in a nourishing way. Too often, too many people have made food solely about education, and, sure, people need to be educated. But some of the most overweight people I have met are some of the most educated when it comes to food and nutrition. So it is not a lack of education that leads someone to polish off a packet of chocolate biscuits after dinner; it is due to biochemistry or emotions, or both. If health professionals fail to address this, the destructive diet mentality that keeps those who struggle with over-eating never feeling that they are good enough is perpetuated.

I believe that the vast majority of people want to be well. They want to be healthy and feel comfortable in their bodies and have great energy. Let's face it: everything is more difficult when you are exhausted. But most people do not know why they do what they do, even when they know what they know. The emotional needs which food meets — knowingly or unknowingly — for millions of people today, coupled with what I describe as the "toxicity factor" of modern life (refer to the liver information elsewhere in this book), the stress factor, the estrogen factor, the thyroid factor, the breathing factor, the gut bacteria factor, and potentially countless more factors that we are yet to discover, all play a major role in every aspect of our wellness.

So when you are struggling to change something that you know in your heart of hearts needs to change (eating too much food, starving yourself, eating too much poor-quality food even though you know better, consuming too much alcohol, too much coffee, too much TV, getting stuck in a social media time-warp), instead of looking at it as something you need to "give up", look at what this is giving you. And then seek out other non-health-harming ways to obtain that feeling. We are governed by how we feel, not the "thing". We are looking to that substance or action to lead us to feel in a certain way. Identify the feeling, and then find it in other ways.

> ## Instead of looking at it as something you need to 'give up', look at what this is giving you.

Use the worksheet on page 219 to help you gain personal insights

Acknowledge
your fears

——

If you feel that stress is really at the heart of your low energy, then I urge you to consider this. Yes, stress can be incredibly energy-zapping, particularly chronic stress. Yet the real word for stress is fear. Whatever you are stressed about — anything at all — it is usually what you are frightened of.

Peel back the layers on what you perceive are your stresses — running late, for example — and see what's really there. See what you are actually afraid of. Of being a failure, of being seen as lazy, of people not liking you, of letting others down...

For most people, when they peel it all back, their fear is that they are not loved, or that there will be a loss of love. Everything — and I mean everything — comes back to avoiding rejection and obtaining or maintaining love. I don't know how else to say it. People think the opposite of stressed is relaxed or calm.

I say it is trust.

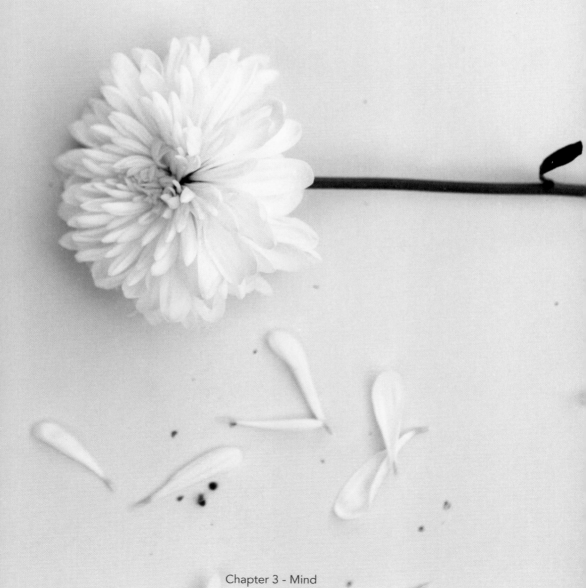

Condition your calm

It doesn't seem to matter if we have two things to do or 200, we can be in a pressing rush to do it all; yet for many of us it rarely feels like we are in control, or on top of any of it. In fact, our desire to control even the smallest details of life can be part of the challenge.

You only have to look around to notice that many people are struggling with achieving a sense of calm in their lives. Many people feel overwhelmed, stressed and rushed to the point that their physical and emotional health is affected. The reasons for this are numerous — the pace of modern life, the responsibilities of full-time work and raising a family, looking after grandchildren, or running a demanding business, to name a few — but sometimes we bring it on ourselves. The rush starts and finishes with ourselves. After all, we are busy with what we say yes to. Many women have a tendency to want to be all things to all people, and we can find it difficult to say no. But what this rush is communicating to our bodies is changing the face of women's health as we know it, from worsening premenstrual syndrome to irritable bowel syndrome, from losing our tempers with loved ones or colleagues to feeling like we just can't cope with day-to-day demands, let alone achieve our goals.

In the rush of it all, how can you slow down? Small steps can result in large pay-offs when it comes to your sense of calm, your happiness and your sense of wellbeing.

Here are some tips to get you started on how you can condition your calm:

ADDRESS YOUR CAFFEINE CONSUMPTION

In a world with a significant coffee culture, it is no wonder many people have become somewhat addicted to their daily caffeine fix. However, what is often not considered is the impact that excessive amounts of caffeine can have on our already stressed/amped-up nervous systems. Caffeine drives the production of adrenalin, one of our stress hormones, which is also why it makes many of us initially feel alert and energized. The flip-side is that often it can lead to anxious feelings and further perpetuate the biochemical effects of the stress we are already encountering. Green tea is a wonderfully uplifting beverage to consume, in place of coffee or to help you reduce your caffeine consumption. It contains an amino acid called "l-theanine", which boosts energy levels but also helps to keep us calm. Packed full of antioxidants, green tea is a health-promoting alternative to coffee, with much less caffeine.

TAKE A NAP

It's as if too many people have become too "proud" to take naps — "they are for the weak", "how could I possibly have time to sleep during the day!" In fact, they are absolutely invigorating and need to be encouraged. Instead of reaching for another coffee or tea, recharge your batteries properly. Taking a 15-minute nap is a great way to reset your nervous system and wake up feeling energized. While this may not be practical at work, it's a wonderful thing to do on the weekend. Research into populations who live well and live long has shown that the one thing they all have in common is that they regularly nap!

CREATE A TECH-FREE ZONE IN
YOUR HOME FOR ONE DAY A WEEK

It is hard to imagine a world without the sounds of cellphones and emails — but it is possible. Take a break from technology once a week (preferably on the weekend), and feel your nervous system start to calm: it can happen almost immediately. Allow yourself the time to just be. Schedule this at least once a week, and become stricter with yourself around the use of your phone, laptop or tablet in the evening.

RE-EVALUATE YOUR TO-DO-LIST
AND SCHEDULE TASKS INSTEAD

How many of the items you have listed on your to-do list need to be done by you? How many can be done by a colleague, a family member or a friend? How many of them need to be done at all? How many of them need to be done now? One of the ways we can create more calm in our lives on a daily basis is to re-evaluate our workload, prioritize and schedule.

LEARN HOW TO SAY NO (GENTLY)

If this feels really uncomfortable for you, make a list of what energizes you and what drains you. If the "drains me" list is longer, start by cutting back on one of those activities or obligations. If that's not possible, then whenever possible seek help, from a friend, a loved one or a colleague. You show strength, courage and honesty when you can ask for help.

PUT YOUR LEGS UP THE WALL

A great way to help you breathe diaphragmatically is to lie on your back with your legs up the wall. Lie in this position for 5–10 minutes and focus on your breath. Place a folded towel under your back or bottom for support if you like. Take 10 minutes to fully relax into this pose; it's especially delicious with some soothing music. Diaphragmatic breathing helps to activate the part of the nervous system responsible for eliciting calm feelings.

CREATING CALM THROUGH MOVEMENT

When you feel like you have a one-way ticket on the stress express, it's not uncommon to be drawn to high-intensity exercise in an effort to "sweat it out". While that most definitely works for some people, it might not work for you, plus, in the long term, high-intensity exercise can drive processes inside of us that drive oxidation and inflammation; essentially, the way we age from the inside out. When you have been in a constant state of stress, you tend to neglect or even avoid calming activities. Consider enrolling in a meditation course and committing to do so with a friend, or go to a restorative yoga class. Incorporate a breath-focused practice in your life, whether that is mediation, yoga, t'ai chi, pilates or even just 10–15 minutes every day where you focus on slow belly-breathing. This is one of the best ways to switch off your stress response. This isn't being indulgent: it's incredibly necessary for your health.

LISTEN TO YOUR BODY

If you feel like cancelling plans, snuggling up on the couch and reading a book, do it — and enjoy it! Far too often we ignore our own intuition about what we need in each moment; instead, we feel obligated to carry through on our original plans. Make a conscious effort to tune into and act on this: you will feel so much better for it.

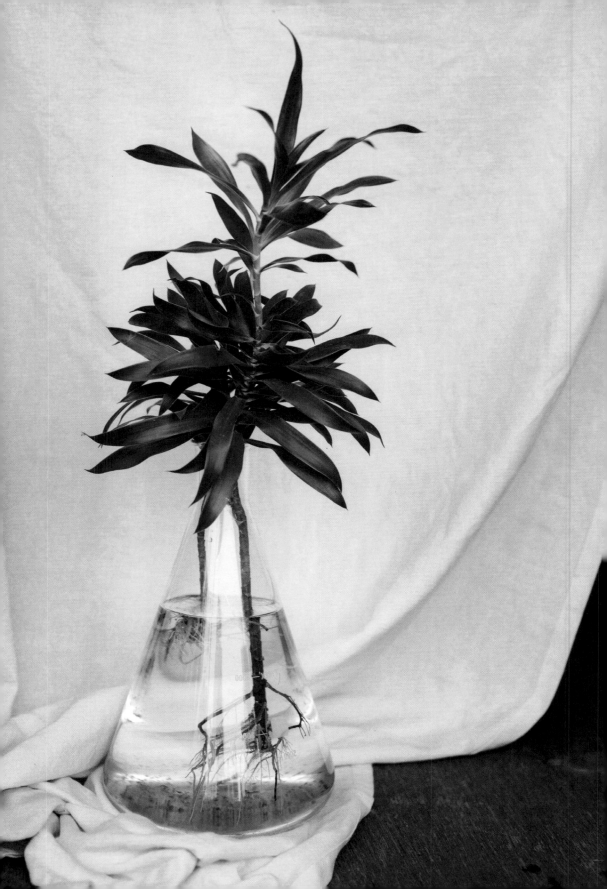

Try something new

To change your health and energy, you have to change something or multiple things. You can't just do what you always do. That is creating how you feel now. Instead of being frustrated by, or simply tolerating your fatigue or your congested skin, for example, consider the parts of your body or the symptoms that irritate or sadden you as simply messengers asking you to eat, drink, move, think, breathe, believe or perceive in a new way.

See them as the gifts that they are.

Think about a part of your body that brings you a source of frustration.

Write it here: ....

For example, you may write "pimples on my face".

Now take some time to reflect on your frustration, across each area listed below, to uncover what your body might be trying to encourage you to do differently.

EAT

Think about a food you've eaten lately, did that make the frustration you listed above worse or better? Could you eat in a more helpful way? What foods might assist you to get rid of your frustration? Capture your insights below.

....

....

....

....

....

....

DRINK

Are you drinking in a way that supports your health or could your current frustration be trying to ask you to drink differently? It could be what you're drinking, when you're drinking or simply that you're not drinking enough. Capture your insights below.

THINK

Our thoughts are incredibly powerful. How could you think differently and in doing this how might this impact the frustration you currently feel?

BREATHE

When was the last time you noticed how you were breathing? Could the way you're breathing be influencing your frustration? Capture your thoughts below.

BELIEVE

What do you truly believe about yourself? What do you truly believe about your present frustration? Do you believe that you deserve great health and energy?

PERCEIVE

Currently how do you perceive your frustration? Do you see it as a "flaw" or an "imperfection" or do you see it as a message from your body that it needs you to make some different choices?

If I don't do it...

IT WON'T GET DONE

How often do you hear yourself say this? It's usually in reference to household chores, or to other tasks that require someone to take responsibility. Yet this statement can also offer insight into a shift that a woman has had in her relationships and how she perceives she has to be.

When you work with people for over two decades, you are privileged to hear thousands of stories. And, although the details of people's stories are individual, there are many patterns that are the same. And this is a common one.

If you are in an intimate relationship, whether it is heterosexual or homosexual, there is usually a person with a more feminine essence, and the other person will have a more masculine essence. In its nature, masculine energy is present. It is directed, focused and action-oriented, and there is immense strength in that presence. There is a backbone, which the feminine deeply appreciates, as this allows her to relax. The feminine is free, changeable, flowing. Like the ocean, the native state of the feminine is to flow with great power but in no single direction. The masculine builds canals, dams and boats to get from point A to point B, but the feminine moves in many directions at once. The masculine chooses a single goal and moves in that direction. Like a ship cutting through a vast ocean, the masculine decides on a course and navigates toward a defined destination, while feminine energy itself is undirected but immense, like the wind and deep currents of the ocean, ever-changing, beautiful, destructive and the source of life.

Any time you force yourself — or someone else knowingly or unknowingly drives you — to be more like a ship than an ocean, you are negating your feminine energy. Any time your man talks to you and expects you to analyse your mood and situation to the point of being able to "fix" it, he is talking "masculine" with you. You can do this — you may even be better at it than he is — but it won't make you a happy woman.

A happy woman is a woman relaxed in her body and heart: powerful, unpredictable, deep, potentially wild and destructive, or calm and serene, but always full of life, surrendered to and moved by the great force of her oceanic heart. Women do not become "free" by analysing themselves. They become free by surrendering to love. Not anyone else's love. Their love. They become free by surrendering to the immense flow of love that is native to their core, and by allowing their lives to be moved by this force. It may involve moments of analysis, but primarily it involves deep trust.

The feminine purpose is the flow of love in relationships (intimate, family and friendships). The masculine priority is purpose and direction, but many men and women today have lost touch with what they want and what lights them up, or they believe they can't have it or don't deserve it. If you want more love, bring more love to every situation you encounter. It sounds counter-intuitive, but, whatever you want more of, share it with others. This allows your love and connection, as well as your femininity, to shine.

So when you hear yourself say (whether out loud or in your mind) "If I don't do it, it won't get done", allow that to press a pause button that encourages you to reflect on what's happening. When you first met your partner, in your connection with them, were you free and flexible, or rigid and directed? The more masculine the man, the freer and more flowing you will likely have been. And what was he like? Present, with a backbone? Did he do what he said he would do? Likely. And what about now? If you feel that "If I don't do it, it won't get done", then it may well be that he has stopped being true to his word and following through on what he said he will do. So the less of a backbone he has, the more rigid and action-oriented you become.

If the feminine is located at the North Pole and the masculine at the South Pole, you get polarity. So when one moves to be more like the other and moves away from its native pole, the other one does, too, in an attempt to maintain polarity.

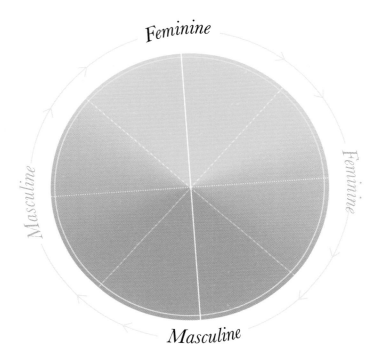

In other words, the more feminine traits the masculine adopts, the more masculine traits the feminine adopts, and vice versa. And neither like their behaviour much when they behave in these ways. The man will say he feels like he can "never win" — in other words, he feels like he can never please her. So he plays computer games or watches sport so he feels like he can win. And she just gets on and does more than her fair share, and silently (or at times outwardly) resents it. And she starts to resent him. In this state, no one has optimal health, as there is tension in the body and the mind. What's more, from this place they start reacting to one another in the light of past experiences, expecting them to be a certain way ("let you down") and so they do.

So how do you begin to undo it? By having an honest conversation about how you feel. Own it that you get tough and harsh (if you do), and allow him the space to do the same: allow him to own that he feels indecisive and that he procrastinates. If you need to embrace masculine traits at work — which most of us do, and are entirely capable of doing so — you will need 30 minutes as a transition from work to home, to return to your feminine. Restorative practices and feminine rituals can assist with this. Listen to music on the way home, or simply change your clothes. Light a candle if that appeals. If you have children, you might ask your partner to play with them while you have your 30-minute break, and at first he may resist this and feel that it's unfair, as he's worked all day, too. But the difference in how you feel, and therefore your behaviour if you get this space, will help him to appreciate how much benefit everyone gains from this space.

You also have to not do all of the things all of the time. You have to sit back sometimes to allow him to step up. When I suggest this to women, most of them say "but he just won't do it". But you don't know until you have genuinely tried to shift back your polarity. Do you really think he values himself when he isn't contributing? Most men place much of their worth on taking action. It makes them feel good.

There is no easy answer and there is no one-size-fits-all solution to this. But both of you recognizing that this is occurring is certainly the first step. Express your needs and really listen to your partner's, and work on creating a way forward that allows both of you to more genuinely be who you really are.

Your health and happiness will love you for it.

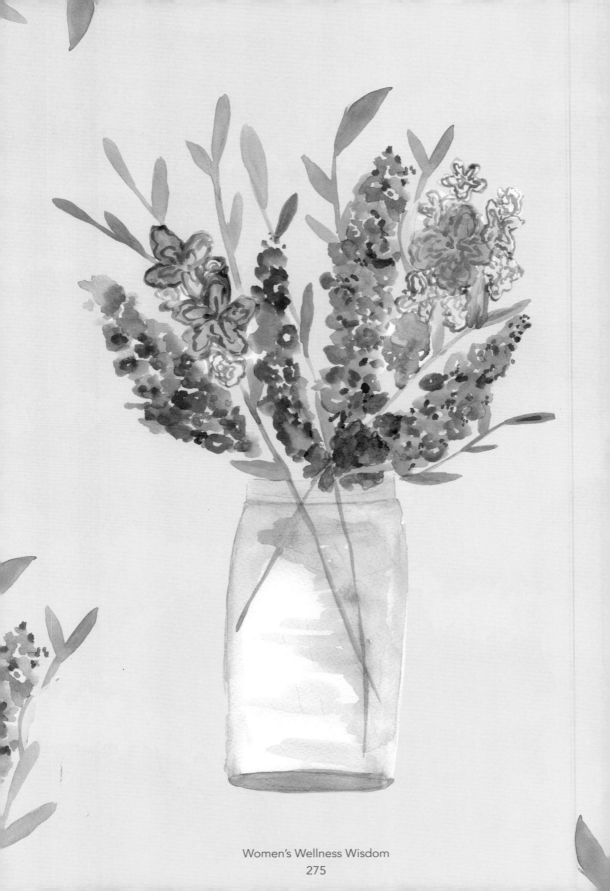

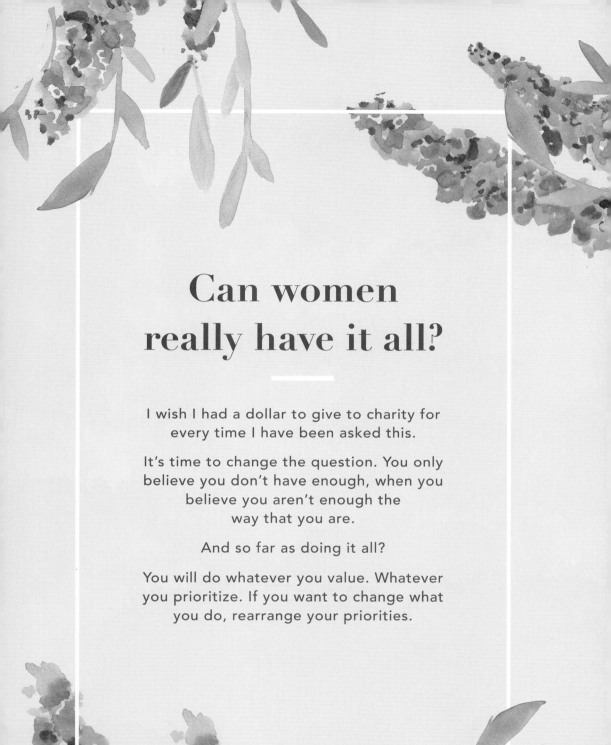

Can women really have it all?

I wish I had a dollar to give to charity for every time I have been asked this.

It's time to change the question. You only believe you don't have enough, when you believe you aren't enough the way that you are.

And so far as doing it all?

You will do whatever you value. Whatever you prioritize. If you want to change what you do, rearrange your priorities.

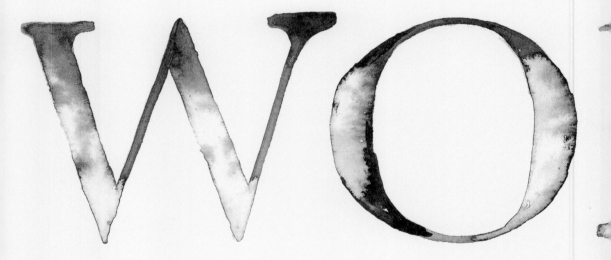

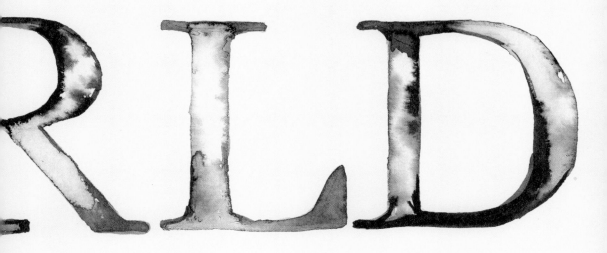

Always maintain an awareness of the big picture of your world. Everything we do or say has an impact. Every choice we make is casting a vote for the characteristics of the type of world that we want. Be aware of the ripple effect you generate through your choices and words. Live and be the change that you want to see in the world.

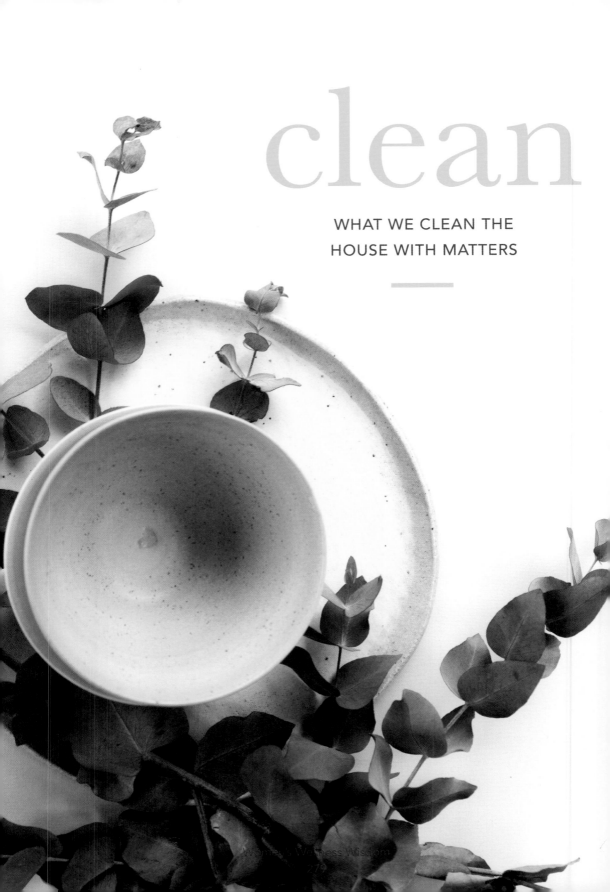

clean

WHAT WE CLEAN THE
HOUSE WITH MATTERS

What we clean the house with matters, not only because the ingredients can disrupt our endocrine systems and add to our liver-load, but also the water that goes down the plug-hole can end up in the ocean or rivers or penetrating the soil.

All of this stays in the food chain, and can come back to enter our body in the future based on what we eat and drink. Think more endocrine disruption and liver-loading.

Did you know that the average home is filled with thousands of synthetic chemicals? And only a small percentage of these chemicals have been thoroughly tested for safety. Very few have had long-term safety studies done, as they haven't been around long enough for us to do so. It's crazy considering how often we are exposed to these chemicals, and how little we know about their effects on our health and the environment. Of those that have been studied, at least 150 common household chemicals have been associated with cancer, psychological disturbances, allergies, gastrointestinal disorders and various health issues.

Cleaning agents contribute a substantial amount to the toxic chemical load in our homes. Many contain solvents, ammonia, formaldehyde, phthalates and ethanolamine. With so many viable natural cleaning solutions now available, how could the potential (and known) risks of these toxins ever be worth a bleached-clean home?

There are numerous reputable companies now producing highly effective, ecologically safe household cleaning products. Seek them out! Plus, many essential oils can mimic the results of chemical cleaners. They can dissolve grease, brighten stains or kill mould spores, but without the potential health concerns. I cannot encourage you enough, as part of your wellness plan, to overhaul or phase-out the use of ordinary cleaning products from your home and embrace the brilliance — for human health and planet — of the myriad eco-friendly cleaning solutions that are natural, non-toxic, simple and effective.

Time management

A GAME-CHANGING SKILL FOR A MORE SPACIOUS AND ENERGIZED LIFE

What do experts in their fields do to maintain and better support their energy? To understand this better, for me it meant conducting interviews and reading a lot.

Here's a condensed version of what I learned.

A time-management strategy I was taught many years ago involved dumping everything on my plate into a notebook (or later an app), and then coding it A1, A2, A3, B1, B2, C1... etc, based on how high up my priority list it was. This is helpful to some degree. But do you really think that the people in the world who have to be the most time-efficient, and juggle more than we could ever wrap our heads around, use such a system? Kevin Kruse, who writes about whole-hearted leadership and researches time management and productivity, interviewed over 200 billionaires, Olympians, straight-A students and entrepreneurs. He asked them to give him their best time-management and productivity advice. And none of them ever mentioned a to-do list.

There are three big problems with a straightforward to-do list. Firstly, a to-do list does not account for time. If you have a long list of tasks, you tend to tackle those that can be completed quickly in a few minutes, leaving the longer items left not done. You want to tick items off to feel good, to feel like you have achieved. Fair enough, but have you actually nailed what needs doing?

Kruse found research from the company iDoneThis indicated that 41 per cent of all to-do list items are never completed. And when I wrote *Rushing Woman's Syndrome*, I found that this bothers more women (and possibly men; although I didn't survey men)

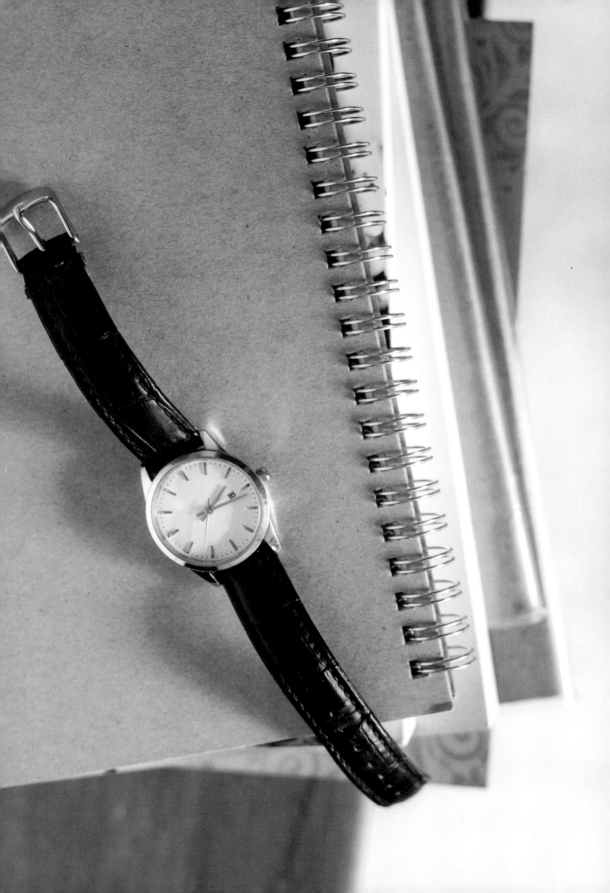

than it does not. And if a to-do list with items that are not all crossed-off does bother you, this is a sure-fire way to make stress hormones. And as you now know, this can be a fast and furious road to poor health and fatigue.

Secondly, a to-do list does not distinguish between which tasks are the most urgent and important. Once again, our impulse is to fight the urgent and ignore the important. For example, how many people put off having medical tests that are actually extremely important? Or going for a walk, because you would have to have your head buried in the sand for your whole life to not know that moving your body is critical to your health, energy and longevity. Let's face it, if exercise were a pill we'd all be taking it. A colonoscopy and a walk may be in different leagues, but they might just be incredibly important, yet most people put them off.

Thirdly, to-do lists contribute to stress. In what is known in psychology as the "Zeigarnik effect", unfinished tasks contribute to intrusive, uncontrolled thoughts. It's no wonder so many people feel so overwhelmed in the day, and then fight insomnia at night.

When you explore time-management research, including Kruse's, one consistent theme keeps coming up: highly productive people do not work from a to-do list — they live and work from their calendar.

When you have a huge number of tasks that need completing in a day and/or you have other people relying on you, the only way the ultra-busy can pull it all off is to prioritize and keep a schedule that for some of them is almost minute-by-minute.

Other people in the time-management research, when asked to reveal their secret for getting so much done, included: "If it's not in my calendar, it won't get done. But if it is in my calendar, it will get done. I schedule out every 15 minutes of every day to conduct meetings, review materials, write and do any activities I need to get done. And while I take meetings with just about anyone who wants to meet with me, I reserve just one hour a week for these 'office hours'." Another quote was: "I simply put everything on my schedule. That's it. Everything I do on a day-to-day basis gets put on my schedule. Thirty minutes of social media — on the schedule. Forty-five minutes of email management — on the schedule. Catching up with my virtual team — on the schedule."

The bottom line on much of what I read was as obvious as this is: if it doesn't get scheduled, it doesn't get done. So here are some suggestions from all I read if you feel that your biggest health- and energy-zapper is a sense of being overwhelmed and having poor time management — a constant case of the feeling that there are not enough hours in the day. The ideas won't be everyone's cup of tea, as I know that scheduling every last thing can feel tedious and creativity-killing. It can also feel like there will be a great big lack of spontaneity in your life if you embrace such an existence. And I personally get that. The only thing is, if you want to feel more spaciousness in your life, try scheduling even three days out of seven and see how that creates a far more spacious headspace for creativity and innovation to flow. Many people who initially resist scheduling, due to the perceived lack of creativity it will allow, find that they become more creative, plus they are more present with what they are doing. When you are playing with your children, how often do you think about everything that's not done? Yet if you think of this while playing and it is scheduled, you can relax knowing that the time will come to do that task, allowing you to be more present with the playing.

The bottom line is if it doesn't get scheduled it doesn't get done.

For some of you, scheduling every day will end your to-do list, you'll get more done, and the energy-zapping stress will lessen as you have a sense that you are handling what's on your plate.

Here are some tips from some heart-centred entrepreneurs, who also happen to be some of the busiest people, making such a difference in the world!

- time-management research results suggest that you make the default event duration in your calendar 15 minutes. Most systems automatically schedule new events for 30 or 60 minutes' duration. Highly productive people only spend as much time as is necessary for each task. When your default setting is 15 minutes, you will automatically discover that you can fit more tasks into each day

- try time-blocking the most important things in your life, first. Don't let your calendar fill up randomly by accepting every request that comes your way. First, get clear on your personal and work priorities and pre-schedule sacred time-blocks for these items. That might include two hours each morning to work on the strategic plan your boss asked you for, or 20 minutes of time for meditation every morning. Mark your calendar to include time-blocks for things like exercise, a date night or other items that align with your core life values

- time-management principles suggest that you schedule everything. Instead of checking emails every few minutes, schedule three times a day to do this. Instead of writing "call Sarah" on your to-do list, put it on your calendar or establish a recurring time-block each afternoon to "return phone calls"

What is scheduled actually gets done. Would you feel less stressed and more productive if you could rip up your to-do list and work from your calendar instead?

Consider utilizing this as a health-enhancing, energy-creating resource in your life.

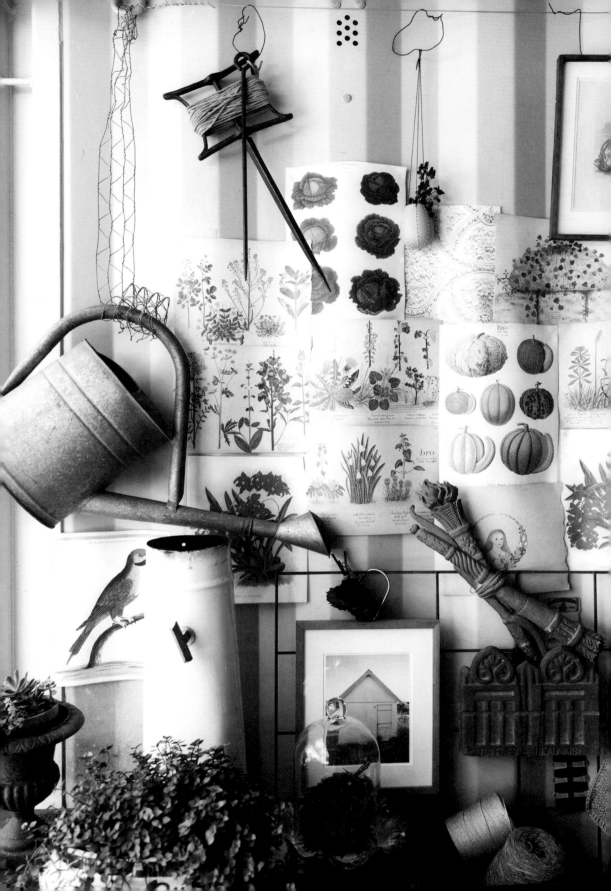

So many screens ...

WHAT IS THIS DOING TO YOU?

Light can disrupt the messages the body is supposed to receive to wind down and fall asleep. Certainly a major change in how many people live has occurred with the use of back-lit devices and the time we spend in front of screens, the television included.

In 2013, humans in the First World spent, on average, three hours a day in front of the television. To put this in perspective, if you watched this amount of television daily and lived to be 75 years of age you would have spent nine years of your life in front of a television. Really ponder that. Nine years of your entire and very precious life. Doesn't that seem excessive? And boring? And not only do people report feeling tired after watching a screen for extended periods, but research has clearly shown that this occurs.

Another challenge with the excessive use of screens, and back-lit devices in particular, is due to the blue light they emit. There is a lot of evidence that blue light, emitted by smart phones, tablets, laptops and many other electronic devices, is impacting on the quantity and quality of the sleep we are getting. Darkness is a natural cue to our bodies that it's time for sleep, but too many people are circumventing it by staring at bright screens for hours after the sun has gone down.

Blue light tells our brain that it isn't time to sleep. There are about 30,000 cells inside your eye that are reactive to the wavelength of light which would be considered blue. This wavelength of light hits the eye cells and drives them to send a signal to an area of the brain known as the suprachiasmatic nucleus, and tells it to turn off melatonin production. Yet, as you probably know, melatonin is the key that starts the sleep engine.

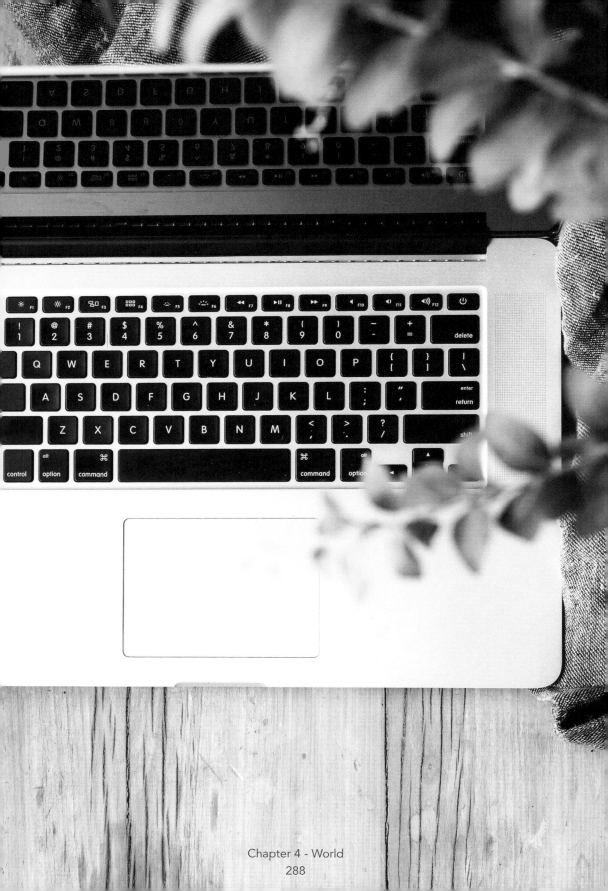

In the past 50 years, research shows that there has been a decline in average duration and quality of sleep, with adverse consequences on our general health. For example, Harvard University undertook a study that assessed two groups: half of the study participants read a printed (paper) book for four hours before bedtime for five consecutive nights, while the other group read a light-emitting ebook reader for the same period. The patients using the ebook reader showed suppressed levels of melatonin. On average, they took longer to fall asleep and displayed significantly less rapid eye movement (REM) sleep (deep sleep) than the group reading printed books.

Unsurprisingly, the ebook group reported feeling more tired in the morning, despite having the same duration of sleep as the other group.

In addition to the impacts on sleep, excessive blue light has also been linked to headaches and eye strain and worsening eyesight, with suggestions that prolonged exposure may cause damage to the retina and contribute to what is referred to as "age-related macular degeneration", which can lead to loss of vision.

Darkness is a natural cue to our bodies that it's time to sleep. Blue light tells our bodies that it isn't time to sleep.

We need to know about the potential impact of excessive, prolonged exposure to blue light, so we can make informed lifestyle choices … even more so if our sleep quality is poor. For when we wake up tired, so many of our daily choices are affected — think food choices, caffeine, the way we react to others and the circumstances of our day.

Strategies to consider incorporating into your lifestyle to promote better sleep and vision include:

1

Avoid using back-lit devices for two hours before bed.

2

Dim the lights in your environment two hours before you want to go to sleep.

3

If you read (long) articles on a back-lit device, look up and focus on something in the distance every few minutes, to allow the muscles that support good vision to not be stuck in one place for too long.

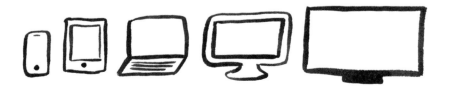

HOW DO YOUR SCREEN CHOICES LEAD YOU TO FEEL?

When I am looking to help people make sustained changes to their lives, I first seek to understand what feelings or experiences the behaviour they want to change (quite often it is food-related) gives them. It might be "relaxation" or "to distract myself from my problems" or "fun". So if all I were to do was suggest that you change something — in this case, time spent in front of the television — and I didn't find out what gives you the feeling you are seeking from the screen, and help you find another way to obtain that, then you would most likely return to your original behaviour.

According to research, television viewing may not be as relaxing as you think. Yes, to an extent television can be relaxing, but only while you watch a show you enjoy. Once the show ends, people report feeling depleted of their energy and as having lower levels of alertness.

Recent research found that study participants commonly reflected that television had somehow "absorbed or sucked out their energy", leaving them depleted. They said they had more difficulty concentrating after viewing than before, and that, in contrast, they rarely indicated such difficulty after reading. After playing sports or engaging in hobbies, people reported improvements in mood, yet after watching television, people's moods were about the same or worse than before they began viewing.

In addition, it has been found that people who watch a lot of television are more likely to be anxious and less happy than people who watch less television in situations where they have nothing to do.

But don't go putting your television out on the side of the road for the rubbish collection just yet. Small amounts can be okay for you, depending on the topics you are watching. In small doses, some studies say it can even be beneficial. Problems with energy, however, begin to emerge when television viewing becomes excessive. And the three hours or more a day, mentioned above, is excessive.

Some of us are so unaware of how much time we spend in front of screens that it can help to keep a diary for a week to track your viewing habits. Placing a limit on how much television you watch is also a good idea. Try your best to be selective about the shows you watch rather than just watching whatever happens to be on.

And next time you are in front of the television, ask yourself this: are you watching television because you really want to, or because you feel bored or lonely, or perhaps you have lost touch with other ways of relaxing? If these last two are the case, brainstorm all of the things you could do instead of watching television.

For instance, you could:
- create some real-food snacks to have ready for the days ahead
- read a book
- go for a walk
- meditate
- phone a friend you haven't spoken with for a while
- watch your children sleep
- start expanding on a new idea you have had
- plan a trip away.

By engaging in more active or restorative tasks, you may notice that your energy levels increase, and you are also more likely to feel happier, too.

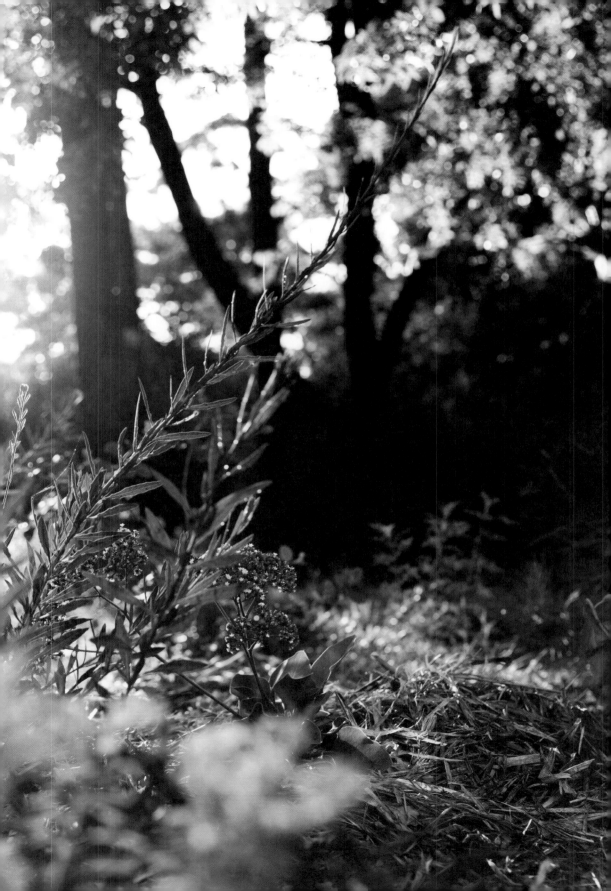

Living longer

WHAT ARE THE "BLUE ZONES" TEACHING US?

We can learn much from illness and the disease processes, sure. Of course this is important so that we can look to prevent and also treat conditions. Yet what is too often overlooked are those who are doing it well. Living in a way that affords them a level of health, beyond that enjoyed by the majority of people: longevity coupled with great physical and mental capabilities, allowing humans to live well to ripe old ages. What can we learn from these people and incorporate more of into our own lifestyles, so that we, too, can live long and live well? Success leaves clues, and Blue Zone research is exploring the lessons the world's longest-lived people are offering us.

Most people living in Blue Zones enjoy physical activity incorporated naturally into their daily lives, like gardening or walking. A sense of purpose is also very strong, such as caring for grandchildren or civic volunteering. They report low stress levels and have a slower pace of life, and there are certainly strong family and community connections. Their way of eating is typically characterized by moderate caloric intake (meaning they don't eat large meals), with their food mostly from plant sources.

Dan Buettner, the lead researcher of the Blue Zone work, shares these "Power 9" lessons as the main traits of the Blue Zone populations.

POWER 9

---

1. Move naturally:

The world's longest-lived people don't pump iron or run marathons. Instead, their environments nudge them into moving without thinking about it.

2. Purpose:

Why do you wake up in the morning? Knowing your sense of purpose is worth up to seven extra years of life expectancy.

3. Down shift:

Stress leads to chronic inflammation, associated with every major age-related disease. The world's longest-lived people have routines to shed that stress.

4. Eighty per cent rule:

"Hara hachi bu" — the Okinawans say this mantra before meals as a reminder to stop eating when their stomachs are 80 per cent full.

5. Plant slant:

The cornerstone of most centenarian diets? Beans. They typically eat meat, mostly pork, only five times per month.

6. Wine at 5:

Moderate drinkers outlive non-drinkers, especially if they share those drinks with friends.

7. Belong:

Attending faith-based services four times per month — no matter the denomination — adds up to 14 years of life expectancy.

8. Loved ones first:

Centenarians put their families first. They have kept aging parents and grandparents nearby, committed to a life partner and invested in their children.

9. Right tribe:

The world's longest-lived people chose, or were born into, social circles that support healthy behaviours.

From: www.bluezones.com

I would like to add that many of the Blue Zone populations have naps!

During the upper Paleolithic period of human history, which was roughly 50,000BC to 10,000BC, the average human life expectancy at birth was 33. By the year 1900, US life expectancy was 46 for men, and 48 for women. Today, it is 76 and 81, respectively. During the 52,000 years between our Paleolithic ancestors and the dawn of the twentieth century, life expectancy rose just 15 years. In the past 114 years, it has increased by 30 years for men, and 33 years for women.

Considering all of the above, then, what lessons from the Blue Zone populations are you keen to embrace or emulate in some way? We want longevity, sure, but we also want a high level of wellness with those years, rather than reliance on others as we have lost the ability to move or function or think for ourselves.

We need to evolve our lifestyle choices to better support the years that are on offer to us.

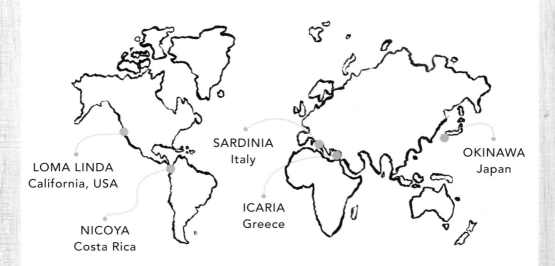

LOMA LINDA
California, USA

NICOYA
Costa Rica

SARDINIA
Italy

ICARIA
Greece

OKINAWA
Japan

AN AWARENESS OF

Privilege

In my practice and women's health weekends, I have been privy to some horrendous experiences that people have endured. The resilience of the human spirit never ceases to break my heart wide open and blow my mind. I have also witnessed what are comparably little things that frustrate, sadden and exhaust people. On top of that I have gained an appreciation of the immense privilege in many people's lives — the privilege of having your basic needs met, when today still too many people in the world don't have this. And amongst all of that, I have witnessed many with such privilege who have been unable to see their lives this way, for a multitude of reasons. And two of those reasons are exhaustion and fear.

You may have created a life where all of your basic needs are met, and then on top of that you have a full-time job, you are continuing education, you have three children and a partner, a house that needs cleaning, planes you have to catch on time, aging parents who need your help... and that is just the tip of the iceberg of your responsibilities and tasks. In such a space, if you cannot see the gift and the immense beauty in all of that — even amidst the chaos — then you are missing out on this extraordinary life you have created. Some of you can't see it this way. Some of you know this and it devastates you. For others, it elicits major feelings of guilt.

And when you complain to me about how hard your (privileged) life is — with all of the above in it — I get it, but I also know you don't really mean that. What I take you to mean is that it is hard to take care of the people you want to take care of with the depth of care you want to demonstrate, and still have something — some energy — left over for you, to do the things that you

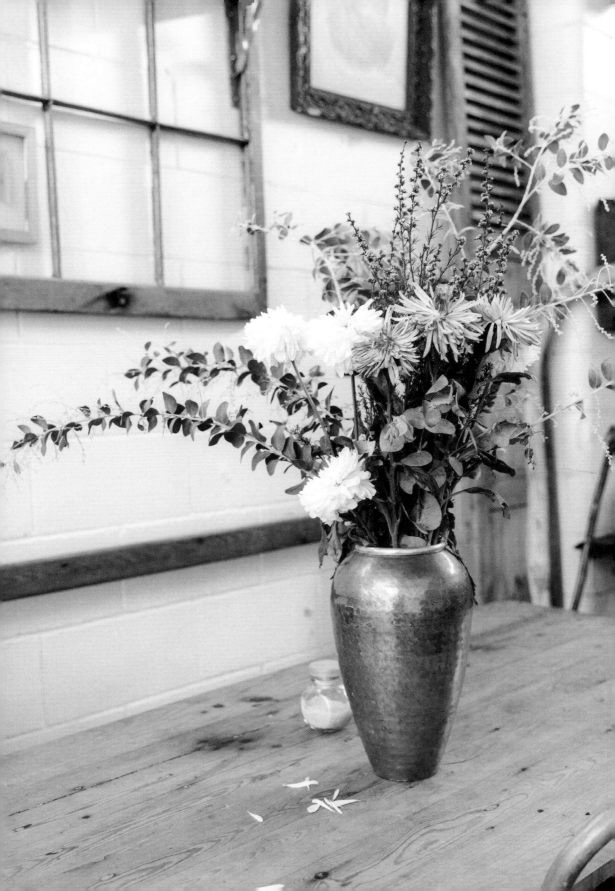

want to do or to simply be, instead of dragging yourself around (whether you let people see this part of you or not) wondering "When is it going to be my turn?" Pretending to have it all together is exhausting in itself. Wondering "When am I going get to do what I want to do?" Worrying constantly about what others think of you. Or you could take a leaf from Oprah's book — remembering that she hasn't always been the Oprah you know her to be today, but has the immense pain of her past — when she suggests you "do what you have to do until you can do what you want to do". Very few situations are permanent.

But if you had good energy and knew that you were enough the way that you are, you would be able to deeply appreciate how extraordinary this incredible life you have created actually is. You would get to enjoy your life instead of feeling like it is hard. For if you have energy, if you have a spacious feeling about a life like this, and a calm and grateful heart — even if what you have to do in a day doesn't change — you enjoy your life and you are a force for good.

When you fight with what is — the fact that you have a mortgage and bills and a demanding job, and challenges with your children and family, and people who need you — when you resist what is, you create a stress so deep within you that you no longer recognize the attitude you show up with every day.

If you had good energy and knew that you were enough the way that you are, you would be able to deeply appreciate how extraordinary this incredible life you have created actually is.

And how you have become saddens you. And the never-ending stress utterly exhausts you.

The biggest obstacle to taking a bigger perspective on life is that our emotions capture and blind us — the anger, the rage, the frustration, the disappointment, the sadness... The more sensitive we become to the blinding capacity of our emotions, the more we realize that when we start getting angry or denigrating ourselves or craving things we don't have in a way that leads us to feel miserable, we begin to shut down. It is like sitting on top of a mountain with the most exquisite view laid out before your eyes, yet you have wrapped yourself in black-out curtains.

You can experiment with this. You can go and sit where there is an amazing view. And the first hit is usually "Wow!" and your mind opens. Yet if you sit there long enough, you will start to worry about something. Then you realize that it feels as though everything is closing in and getting very small. We all do this all day, every day. The skill is to catch ourselves and come back to the view, to the beauty, to be open to the big picture. Do this moment after moment after moment.

Which do you think fosters greater energy? The opening or the closing? The "wow" or the worry? I am not denying that there aren't things to be concerned about; I am simply wanting to offer you a new perspective that encourages you to be open to wonder. To the wonder and gift of life, with all of its messiness and chaos and unpredictability. I can't help but encourage you again to embrace uncertainty, for some of the most beautiful chapters in our lives won't have a title until much later.

To paraphrase Viktor Frankl, we must never forget that we may also find meaning in life when confronted with a hopeless situation, when facing a fate that cannot be changed...

When we are no longer able to change a situation, we are challenged to change ourselves.

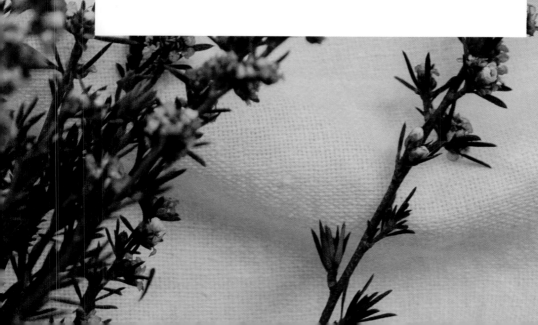

Acknowledgements

Hugest thanks to the team who helped bring
this beautiful book to life: Maddy, Steph and Kate.
Thanks to the team behind the scenes too:
Kate, Jenny, Georgia and Dee.

Special thanks to Chris for making it all
happen and to Max for his entertainment.
You are all so great at what you do and I really
appreciate you and your care.

And to you the reader, for wanting to
take even better care of yourself.

The world is a better place
because you are in it.

The gift that is life

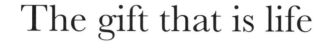

Don't let it take a health crisis or a threat to your mortality to wake you up to make the changes to your lifestyle that you know in your heart you need to make today.

You know when you are having too much of something or too little of something else.

Take care of your inner body systems, to feel and look your best, and to live a long and robust life.

Live each day connected to what a gift life is, how precious you are, and treat yourself accordingly.

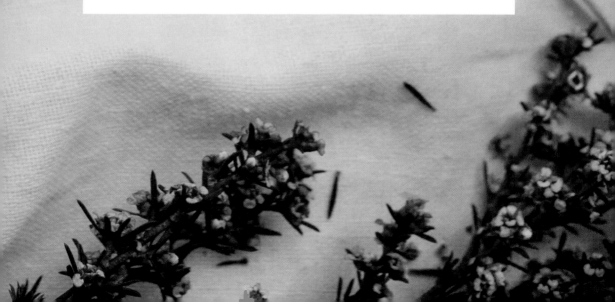

Also by Dr Libby Weaver

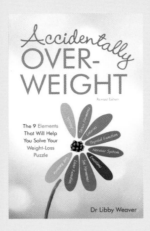

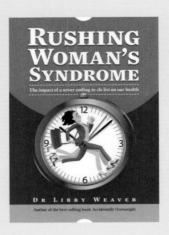

Accidentally Overweight

Accidentally Overweight explores the must-know nine factors essential to successful and sustainable weight loss. They include stress hormones, sex hormones, thyroid function and gut bacteria.

Rushing Woman's Syndrome

Rushing Woman's Syndrome offers you real solutions to both the biochemistry and the emotional patterns of the rush. What you need to do in a day may not change but how you show up can revolutionize how you experience each day and how others experience you.

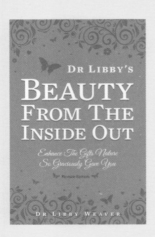

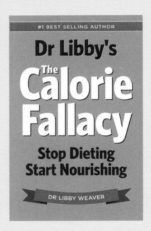

Beauty from the Inside Out

Beauty from the Inside Out is a must-have beauty book for women of all ages. Enjoy radiating your own unique sparkle, from the inside out and learn how everything from nutrients to emotions impacts what is displayed on the outside.

The Calorie Fallacy

This book arms you with the wisdom to stop dieting and depriving yourself and start thriving. Stop dieting and start nourishing and start living with a new freedom with your relationship with food and your body.

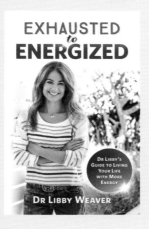

Exhausted to Energized

Everything in life is more difficult when we are exhausted. *Exhausted to Energized* offers you simple but powerful strategies to help liberate you from exhaustion and live a life with more energy.

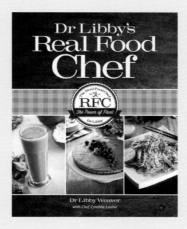

Real Food Chef

The *Real Food Chef* is a beautiful book that will revolutionize the way you are nourished. Filled with delicious and nutrient-dense meals, drinks, snacks and sauces, this book educates and supports you to embrace a real-food way of eating.

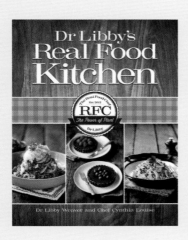

Real Food Kitchen

The *Real Food Kitchen* will inspire you to take better care of yourself with the delicious and nutritious recipes featured. Packed with even more nutritional information as well as recipes that are firm family favourites that have been 'real-food chef-ified', you will love using this beautiful cookbook.

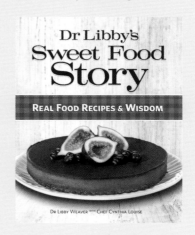

Sweet Food Story

Many people make great food choices for breakfast and lunch, and then at 3 o'clock in the afternoon they feel like someone else has taken over their body, their desire for sweet food can be so intense. The *Sweet Food Story* cookbook was created with this in mind, as a way of educating and supporting you to eat sweet food that serves your health.

REFERENCES AND RESOURCES

After reading *Women's Wellness Wisdom*, you may ask, what's next? I have received and been touched by countless emails from people all over the world saying that they feel like I have read their diary when it comes to describing how they feel in the pages of my books. People tell me that they want more of this type of information, which gives them further insight into their physical and emotional health. I cannot encourage you enough to check out the array of options on my website, including my weekend events and online courses. If you relate to the title *Rushing Woman's Syndrome* but you feel like you don't have time to read the book, you might enjoy the 30-day online *Rushing Woman's Syndrome Quickstart Course* where I guide you on how to retire from being a rushing woman!

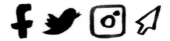

Take a look at the blog, too, at:

www.drlibby.com

I also post health information each weekday on social media. Connect with me there at:

www.facebook.com/DrLibbyLive
www.twitter.com/DrLibbyLive
And on Instagram, find me as @drlibby

———

My passion is to educate and inspire, and to help people change the relationship they have with their bodies and their health, and put the power of choice back in their hands. It is an honour to assist you in your optimal health journey.

I have cited some books and papers in this text and they are listed in full here if further reading in a particular area interests you.

Books, articles and online papers

Bey, L. and Hamilton, M.T. (2003). *Suppression of skeletal muscle lipoprotein lipase activity during physical inactivity: a molecular reason to maintain daily low-intensity activity*. Journal of Physiology 551(Pt 2): 673–682.

Buettner, Dan. (2010). *The Blue Zones*. Washington, D.C.: National Geographic Society.

Hamilton, M.T., Hamilton, D.G., and Zderic, T.W. (2004). *Exercise physiology versus inactivity physiology: an essential concept for understanding lipoprotein lipase regulation*. Exercise Sport Science Review 32(4): 161–166.

www.kevinkruse.com for time management data.

Weaver, Dr Libby. (2011). *Accidentally Overweight*. Auckland: Little Green Frog.

Weaver, Dr Libby. (2012). *Rushing Woman's Syndrome*. Auckland: Little Green Frog.

Weaver, Dr Libby. (2013). *Beauty from the Inside Out*. Auckland: Little Green Frog.

Weaver, Dr Libby. (2014). *The Calorie Fallacy*. Auckland: Little Green Frog.

Weaver, Dr Libby and Tait, Cynthia. (2012). *Dr Libby's Real Food Chef*. Auckland: Little Green Frog.

Weaver, Dr Libby and Tait, Cynthia. (2013). *Dr Libby's Real Food Kitchen*. Auckland: Little Green Frog.

Weaver, Dr Libby and Tait, Cynthia. (2014). *Dr Libby's Sweet Food Story*. Auckland: Little Green Frog.

West Kurz, Susan. (2006). *Awakening Beauty the Dr. Hauschka Way*. New York: Clarkson Potter Publishers.

Whitton, Tracy. (2011). *Stillness Through Movement*. Burleigh, Gold Coast: Tracy Whitton.

CDs

Weaver, Dr Libby. (2012). *Restorative Calm*. Auckland: Little Green Frog.

Whitton, Tracy. (2011). *One With Life*. Burleigh, Gold Coast: Tracy Whitton.

Dr Libby live events and online courses

Available at www.drlibby.com I regularly do speaking tours, so check my website for topics, dates and venues. I also run weekend events that offer participants a wonderful restorative experience coupled with in-depth learning of holistic health: the biochemical, the nutritional and the emotional. The *Beautiful You Weekend* is such a special event.

Online courses and webinars include:

Rushing Woman's Syndrome Quickstart Course

Condition the Calm Course

30 Essential Beauty Gems Course

New Year New You Webinar

Sensational Sleep Webinar

TEDx: *The Pace of Modern Life Versus our Cavewoman Biochemistry* https://www.youtube.com/watch?v=tJ0SME6Z9rw

Understanding the Mysteries and Magic of the Female Body Webinar